DANVILLE

D0380990

A STORY OF THE RED CROSS

GLIMPSES OF FIELD WORK

BY

CLARA BARTON

WITHDRAWN

FOUNDER OF THE AMERICAN NATIONAL RED CROSS
AND PRESIDENT, 1881—1904

NEW YORK
D. APPLETON AND COMPANY
MCMIV

CONTRA COSTA COUNTY LIBRARY

3 1901 04516 2049

COPYRIGHT, 1904, BY

D. APPLETON AND COMPANY

Published, June, 1904

This scarce antiquarian book is included in our special *Legacy Reprint Series*. In the interest of creating a more extensive selection of rare historical book reprints, we have chosen to reproduce this title even though it may possibly have occasional imperfections such as missing and blurred pages, missing text, poor pictures, markings, dark backgrounds and other reproduction issues beyond our control. Because this work is culturally important, we have made it available as a part of our commitment to protecting, preserving and promoting the world's literature.

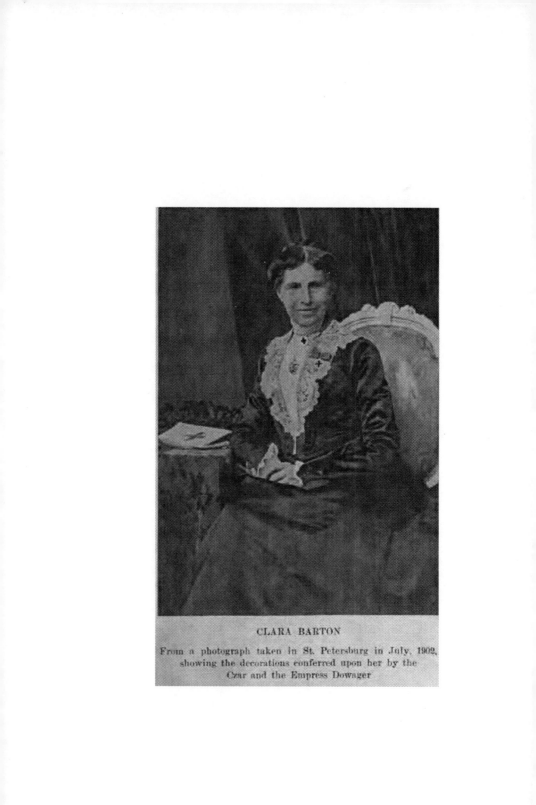

CLARA BARTON

From a photograph taken in St. Petersburg in July, 1902, showing the decorations conferred upon her by the Czar and the Empress Dowager

PREFACE

Since the foundation of the Red Cross in America, many direful calamities have afflicted the country. In each of these visitations the Red Cross has acted in some degree as the Almoner—the distributer and organizer—of the bountiful measures of relief that have been poured out by the American people.

Its work has been accomplished quietly and without ostentation. All the relief has been administered—not as charity—but as God-sent succor to our brothers and sisters who have been overwhelmed by some mighty convulsion of the forces of nature.

The wreckage has been cleared away, the stricken people have been wisely, tenderly, and calmly guided out of panic and despair on to the road of self-help and cooperative effort to restore their shattered homes and broken fortunes; and then the Red Cross has retired as quietly as it came, and

PREFACE

few, outside of the people immediately concerned, have realized the beneficent powers of help and healing that have fallen like a benediction upon the stricken wherever that sacred symbol of humanity has made its way.

It is my thought that a brief account of the work of the Red Cross during the past twenty-five years will be of interest to the American people. In a volume of this size it must of necessity be but a brief outline, sufficient, however, to convey a clear impression of what the Red Cross really means to every individual in this great country of ours.

To the thousands of American men and women whose generous bounty has made the work of the Red Cross possible, to the stricken and distressed who because of it have been helped back to life and hope, and to all the friends of the great, universal humanity which it typifies, this small book is lovingly dedicated.

CLARA BARTON.

GLEN ECHO, MARYLAND,
May 15, 1904.

CONTENTS

CONTENTS

A STORY OF THE RED CROSS

I

EARLY HISTORY

1880-1884

"I have lived much that I have not written, but I have written nothing that I have not lived."

IT was a little blue-eyed girl of ten who sat on a low hassock at my feet, slowly drawing the soft auburn curls between her fingers, when, suddenly lifting her head and looking me earnestly in the face, she exclaimed: "What is the Red Cross? Please tell me about it; I can not understand it."

There was a pleading earnestness in the tone not to be resisted, and laying down my pen I commenced to explain to her the principles, history, and uses of the Red Cross. She listened anxiously, the pretty brow knitted; she seemed more and more perplexed, until, as if a light had broken over her, she exclaimed, half impatiently:

1

"Not that—not that, tell me something it *does*—it and you, I can understand it better then."

A light had broken over me. It was a story the child wanted to illustrate the principle and bring it home to her. A story she must have.

In a half hour she felt that she knew it all and was an ardent devotee even of its principles. But she had given me more than I had given her. Here was food for thought.

For twenty-five years I had labored to explain the principles and uses of the Red Cross; had written enough for a modest library of what it was and what it meant, but, lest I seem egotistical, not a page of what it did. The child had given me an idea that I would for once put into practice, and write a few pages of what the Red Cross had done, leaving principles to present themselves.

I will commence even back of itself.

Forty years ago, before most of you were born, a great war had been fought in America, in which thousands died from battle and hardship, and thousands more still left alive were worn out in the untried and unsystematized efforts at relief that had been made through nearly five years of continuous war. Of these latter, many were women who dragged out weary lives in their own homes, some went to hospitals and retreats for rest and care, and some were sent abroad. One of these latter I knew personally, for, as Patrick would say, " It was me-self."

To me it seemed a hard sentence that our physicians imposed. I had grown to love the country we had so toiled for, and did not want to leave it. Its very woes had made it dear to me. It had quiet once more, and a peace that was not all a peace. It had its early soldier homes, its fast-filling cemeteries, and the tender memory of a martyred President resting over us like a pall. These had come to seem like a heritage to me, and in my weakness I clung to them. Still, the order was obeyed and I went.

Then followed travels in strange and foreign lands, other wars, illness and suffering of my own, until eleven years later I came almost a stranger again to our Government with another work, which I believed to be for its good and the good of our people.

This time I brought the idea of the treaty of

Geneva, asking our Government, at the request of other Governments, to examine and to unite with it, if found desirable. This effort with the Government covers five years of hard, continuous labor, during which was sought the aid of friends known in other years. At the end of this time, by advice of our second martyred President and three members of his historic cabinet—James G. Blaine, William Windom, and Robert T. Lincoln—a national society was formed, known as the Association of the American Red Cross, and, by desire and nomination of President Garfield, I was made its president, and requested to name my officers.

The association was formed during the winter of 1880–'81, with the view on the part of President Garfield of facilitating the adoption of the treaty which he would name in his next message, which message was never written.

Before the message, he, too, had joined the martyred ranks, and his gentle successor, Arthur, filled his chair and kept his promise, and through action of his own executive department the treaty was adopted; indorsed by action of the Senate; proclaimed by the President to our people; later rati-

4

fied by the International Powers in the Congress of Berne, with the pledge to render relief to unfortunate victims of war, and the privilege, by my request, of rendering similar relief to the victims of great national calamities or disasters.

All this had been accomplished by the kindly help of a few personal friends, tireless and unrewarded, and while the news of the accession of the Government of the United States, to the treaty of Geneva, lit bonfires that night (for I cabled it by their request) in the streets of Switzerland, France, Germany, and Spain, a little four-line paragraph in the congressional doings of the day in the *Evening Star*, of Washington, alone announced to the people of America that an international treaty had been added to their rolls.

No personal distinction had been bestowed, no one honored, no one politically advanced, no money of the Government expended, and, like other things of like nature and history, it was left in obscurity to make its own way and live its own hard life.

Thus the spring of 1882 found us—a few people, tired and weak, with five years of costly service, a treaty gained, with no fund, no war nor

5

prospect of any, and no helpful connection with or acknowledgment by the Government.

Soon the news of " Half the State of Michigan on Fire" called us to action on our own laws of civil relief. A little draft on the purse of the new, inexperienced president of the association paved the way for an agent to go to the field. Others generously joined, all reported to our friend and advocate, Senator Omar D. Conger, of Michigan. Some supplies were sent, a society or two formed to provide and forward them. The agents remained until the suffering was relieved, and thus the first field relief work of which we have any record in the United States was commenced.

Meanwhile, I had been asked by the Senate to write the history of the Red Cross, and show the official action taken by our Government on the acceptance of the treaty, which history the Senate would have printed at the Government printing-office. This volume I prepared as requested. A thousand copies were printed for information to the public, to be circulated by the society; but with no frank or other means provided, and with a

6

postage of some ten cents a volume, we were compelled to limit the circulation to the means.

The following year, 1883, a disastrous rise in the Ohio River called for our aid. Dr. J. B. Hubbell, who had been our agent the year before, was called from Michigan University, where he was completing a course, to examine the needs of the inhabitants and take such relief as we could provide. There was little loss of life, and the destruction of property lay largely in the loss of stock, and washing away of the soil, vegetation, and the means of reproduction.

A remarkable provision for this latter loss was made by the gift of Mr. Hiram Sibley, the noted seed dealer of Rochester—who had become associated with the Red Cross, being an old-time friend of the family of its president—of ten thousand dollars' worth of seed, to replant the washed-out lands adown the Mississippi. As the waters rank off the mud immediately baked in the sunshine, making planting impossible after a few days. Accordingly, Mr. Sibley's gift was sent with all haste to our agent at Memphis, and in forty-eight hours, by train and boat, it was distributed in the

7

four States—Tennessee, Arkansas, Louisiana, and Mississippi—and planted for the crops of the coming season.

Besides this generous gift of material, a little money had been raised and sent by the three societies of the Red Cross which had been formed, viz.: Dansville and Syracuse, a few hundreds—something more from the Red Cross at Rochester— always thoughtful and generous, which served to help in the distribution of clothing and supplies promiscuously sent. And at the finish of the work, when every donation had been carefully acknowledged, one thousand dollars and some cents were left in the treasury unexpended.

A cyclone occurring within a few months in Louisiana and southern Alabama, cutting a swath from New Orleans to Mobile, decided us to send eight hundred dollars of this reserve to the secretary of the Red Cross Society of New Orleans, which sum was forwarded by our vice-president, Mr. A. S. Solomons. This left a sum of two hundred dollars and some cents in the treasury with which to commence another field.

This was the commencement of 1883. In May,

at the solicitation of General Butler, then Governor of Massachusetts, I took the superintendence of the Massachusetts Woman's State Prison at Sherborn, at the customary salary of fifteen hundred dollars a year. To this duty the Legislature added, after my arrival, those of secretary and treasurer, without increase of salary, discharging the former incumbent, a man, at three thousand dollars a year. I accepted the new duties, became my own bondsman for ten thousand dollars, by transfer of that amount of bonds from my bankers, Brown Brothers, New York, to the Massachusetts State Treasury at Boston—remaining in charge of the prison until the close of the year, and the retirement of General Butler as Governor.

In the short and interrupted existence of our association—scarce two years—our few official advisers had formed some general regulations, relating to our course of procedure. Realizing that to be of any real service as a body of relief for sudden disasters, we must not only be independent of the slow, ordinary methods of soliciting relief, but in its means of application as well, it was decided:

First. To never solicit relief or ask for contributions.

Second. Not to pay salaries to officers—paying out money only to those whom we must employ for manual labor—and as our officers served without compensation they should not be taxed for dues.

Third. To keep ourselves always in possession of a stated sum of money to commence a field of disaster—this sum to be independent even of the closed doors of a bank which might prevent leaving for a field on a Sunday or holiday.

Fourth. To take this sum of our own, going directly to a field with such help as needed, giving no notice until there, overlooking the field, and learning the extent of the trouble and conditions of the people, making immediate and reliable report to the country through the Associated Press, some of whose officers were our own Red Cross officers as well. These reports would be truthful, unexaggerated, and non-sensational statements that could be relied upon.

Fifth. That if, under these conditions, the people chose to make use of us as distributers of the relief which they desired to contribute to the suf-

10

ferers, we would do our best to serve them while at the field—make report directly to each and all contributors, so far as in our power, and proceed to carry out any directions and apply the relief at hand, in the wisest manner possible, among a dazed and afflicted community.

To inaugurate this method, I, as president, placed a sum of three thousand dollars, free of bank or interest, upon momentary call, at the service of the association. On more than one occasion it has been taken on Sunday, when every bank in the country was closed and charitable bodies were at their prayers. Even the relief of Johnstown was thus commenced. This provision has never for a day been broken. It is as good at this moment as it was in 1883, and from the same source. It may not have been a "business-like" method nor one to be approved by stated boards of directors nor squared by bank regulations. But the foes we had to meet were not thus regulated, and had to be met as they came; and so they always must be if any good is to be accomplished.

Until the Government and society can control the elements, and regulate a spring freshet, a

11

whirlwind or a cyclone, they will find that red tape
is not strong enough to hold their ravages in check.

It was well that these regulations had been for-
mulated and their provisions acted upon, as the
state of our treasury and the conditions immediately following will show.

I returned to Washington upon my retirement
from the superintendence of the State Prison at
Sherborn, accompanied by Dr. Hubbell, who, having completed his university course, had come to
the Red Cross for permanent service. Before we
had even time to unpack our trunks, the news of
the fearful rise of the Ohio River, of 1884, began
to shock the country with its loss of life and property.

I had never been present at a disaster in civil
life. It had never occurred to me that they recurred so frequently. But if by virtue of my
office as president I was liable to be called every
year to preside over and provide for them, it was
essential that I learn my duties experimentally. I
accordingly joined Dr. Hubbell, who had been appointed general field agent, and proceeded to Pittsburg, the headwaters of the rise.

Telegraphing from there to our agents of the Associated Press, we proceeded to Cincinnati, to find the city afloat. Its inhabitants were being fed from boats, through the second-story windows. These conditions were telegraphed. Supplies commenced to flow in, not only from our own societies but from the people of the country. Warehouses were filled, in spite of all we dispensed—but there were four hundred miles of this distress— even to Cairo, where the Ohio, sometimes thirty miles in width, discharged its swollen waters into the Mississippi.

Recognizing this condition lower down the river as the greater need, we transferred our supplies and distribution to Evansville, Ind. Scarcely had we reached there when a cyclone struck the river below, and traveling up its entire length, leveled every standing object upon its banks, swept the houses along like cockle-shells, uprooted the greatest trees and whirled them down its mighty current—catching here and there its human victims, or leaving them with life only, houseless, homeless, wringing their hands on a frozen, fireless shore—with every coal-pit filled with water,

13

and death from freezing more imminent than from hunger.

There were four hundred miles more of this, and no way of reaching them by land. With all our tons of clothing, these people and their homeless little children were freezing. There was but one way—the Government boats had come with rations of food—we too must take to the water.

At eight o'clock in the morning I chartered my first boat, with captain and crew, at sixty dollars per day, to be at once laden to the water's edge with coal—our own supplies to be stored on the upper deck—and at four o'clock in the afternoon, as the murky sun was hiding its clouded face, the bell of the "John V. Troop," in charge of her owner, announced the departure of the first Red Cross relief-boat ever seen on American waters.

I found myself that night with a stanch crew of thirty men and a skilled captain, and a boat under my command. I had never until then held such a command. We wove the river diagonally from side to side—from village to village—where the homeless, shivering people were gathered— called for the most responsible person—a clergy-

14

man if one could be found, threw off boxes of clothing, and hove off coal for a two weeks' supply, and
steamed away to the opposite side, leaving only
gratitude, wonder at who we were, where we came
from, and what that strange flag meant? We
improved every opportunity to replenish our supply of coal, and reached Cairo in five days.

Waiting only to reload, we returned up the
river, resupplied the revived villages of people, too
grateful for words, reaching Evansville at the end
of three weeks, where more supplies than we had
taken awaited us. St. Louis and Chicago had
caught the fever of relief, had arranged societies,
and had asked permission to join our aid. Up to
this time the Mississippi had given no indication
of trouble, but now its great June rise commenced.

The Government boats, by another appropriation, were sent to the Mississippi, and we prepared
to supplement them. Discharging our Ohio
River boat we went to St. Louis by rail and chartered the " Mattie Bell." The Red Cross Societies
of St. Louis and Chicago, under their respective
presidents and officers in charge of them and their
funds, joined us, and together we prepared to feed

15

and rescue the perishing stock—as well as people adown the Mississippi. The animals had never been saved in an overflow; and besides the cruelty of letting them starve by thousands, the loss to the people was irreparable, as the following year must inevitably be replete with idleness and poverty till more stock could be obtained to work with.

We found as commissary at St. Louis, General Beckwith, the historic commissary-general of the old civil war, who had personally superintended the loading of my wagons in Washington, year after year, for the battle-fields of Virginia. He came on board the " Mattie Bell " and personally superintended the lading—clothing, corn, oats, salt, and hay—besides putting upon the Government boats large quantities of supplies which we could not take on at first, and giving us his blessing, watched us steam out on our joint mission; they putting off rations of meat and meal—we supplementing with clothing for the people and feed for the stock. We purchased all we could at cities as we passed, picked our course among the broken levees and roaring crevasses, all the way to New Orleans. The hungry were fed, the naked

16

clothed, and the stock saved. The negro had his mule, and the planter his horses and cattle to carry on his work when the flood should disappear. We had lighter boats, still lighter purses, but lightest of all were the grateful hearts that a kind Providence and a generous people had given to us the privilege of serving.

We discharged the " Mattie Bell " at St. Louis, bidding adieu to the officers of the Red Cross Society, who had rendered most acceptable service to the cause. They had brought their own funds and material—had personally administered them from the decks of the " Mattie Bell," made their own reports, and modestly retired to their home duties, there to await the next call.

Chicago, which had a new Red Cross Society, formed almost for the occasion, through its most worthy and notable representative, Rev. E. I. Galvin, did the same, performing the long journey with us, superintending the distribution of his own relief and making his own report with such convincing power, that societies of no less excellence than the Lend-a-Hand were its outgrowth.

I am thus particular to mention this from the

17

loving gratitude fervently cherished for strong, tender help in the day of small things. Their contributions largely served to run our boat and keep our crew, and with heads, hearts, and hands we struggled as one, to avert the destruction so rife around us.

From St. Louis we crossed over to Evansville, rechartered the "John V. Troop," and put on accumulated supplies. The waters of the Ohio had subsided and the people were returning to the old spots of earth that once had been their home, but there was neither house to live in nor tool to work the land with. We reloaded with pine lumber, ready-made doors, windows, household utensils, stores and groceries, farming utensils, and with a good force of carpenters proceeded up the Ohio once more. The sight of the disconsolate, half-clad farmer waiting on the bank told us where his home had been—and was not.

Three hours' work of our carpenters would put up a one-room house, meanwhile our efficient men and women helpers, among them the best ladies of Evansville, would furnish it with beds, bedding, clothing, provisions for the family, and farming tools ready to go on with the season's work.

Picture, if possible, this scene. A strange ship with a strange flag steaming up the river. It halts, turns from its course, and draws up to the nearest landing. Some persons disembark and speak a few minutes with the family. Then, a half dozen strong mechanics man a small boat laden with all material for constructing a one-room house—floor, roof, doors, windows. The boat returns for furniture. Within three hours the strange ship sails away, leaving a bewildered family in a new and clean house with bed, bedding, clothing, table, chairs, dishes, candles, a little cooking-stove with a blazing fire, all the common quota of cooking utensils, and meat, meal, and groceries; a plow, rake, axe, hoe, shovel, spade, hammer, and nails. We ask few questions. They ask none. The whistle of the " Troop " is as welcome to their ears as the flag to their eyes.

At one of these wrecked villages the entire little hamlet of people stood on our decks. Only four, they said, were left at home, and these were sick. They had selected their lawyer to speak their thanks. No words will ever do justice to the volume of native eloquence which seemed to roll unbidden from his lips. He finished with these sentences:

" At noon on that day we were in the blackness of despair—the whole village in the power of the demon of waters—hemmed in by sleet and ice, without fire enough to cook its little food. When the bell struck nine that night, there were seventy-five families on their knees before their blazing grates, thanking God for fire and light, and praying blessings on the phantom ship with the unknown device that had come as silently as the snow, they knew not whence, and gone, they knew not whither."

When we finished the voyage of relief, we had covered the Ohio River from Cincinnati to Cairo and back twice, and the Mississippi from St. Louis to New Orleans, and return—four months on the rivers—traveled over eight thousand miles, distributed in relief of money and estimated material, one hundred and seventy-five thousand dollars—gathered as we used it.

We left at one point on the Ohio River a well-

lettered cross-board, " Little Six Red Cross Landing "—probably there to this day. The story of
The Little Six might be given in their own little
letter:

WATERFORD, PA., *March 24*, 1884.

DEAR MISS BARTON:

We read your nice letter in the Dispatch and
we would like very much to see that house called
" The Little Six," and we little six are so glad
that we helped six other little children, and we
thank you for going to so much trouble in putting
our money just where we would have put it ourselves. Some time again when you want money
to help you in your good work call on " The Little
Six."

> JOE FARRAR, twelve years old.
> FLORENCE HOWE, eleven years old.
> MARY BARTON, eleven years old.
> REED WHITE, eleven years old.
> BERTIE AINSWORTH, ten years old.
> LOYD BARTON, seven years old.

These children had given a public entertainment
for the benefit of the flood sufferers. They themselves suggested it, planned and carried it out, and

raised fifty-one dollars and twenty-five cents, which they sent to the editor of the Erie Dispatch, asking him to send it " where it would do the most good." The Dispatch forwarded it to the president of the Red Cross, with an account of the entertainment given by " The Little Six."

The entire matter was too beautiful and withal unique, to meet only a common fate in its results. I could not, for a moment, think to mingle the gift of the little dramatists with the common fund for general distribution, and sought through all these weeks for a fitting disposition to make of it, where it would all go in some special manner to relieve some special necessity. I wanted it to benefit some children who had " wept on the banks " of the river, which in its madness had devoured their home.

As we neared that picturesque spot on the Illinois side of the Ohio, known as " Cave-in Rock," we were hailed by a woman and her young daughter. The boat " rounded to " and made the landing and they came on board—a tall, thin, worn woman in tattered clothes, with a good but inexpressibly sad face, who wished to tell us that a package which we had left for her at the town on our way down had never reached her. She was a widow—Mrs. Plew—whose husband, a good river pilot, had died from overwork on a hard trip to New Orleans in the floods of the Mississippi two years before, leaving her with six children dependent upon her, the eldest a lad in his " teens," the youngest a little baby girl. They owned their home, just on the brink of the river, a little " farm " of two or three acres, two horses, three cows, thirty hogs, and a half hundred fowls, and in spite of the bereavement, they had gone on bravely, winning the esteem and commendation of all who knew them for thrift and honest endeavor. Last year the floods came heavily upon them, driving them from their home, and the two horses were lost. Next the cholera came among the hogs and all but three died. Still they worked on; and held the home. This spring came the third flood. The water climbed up the bank, crept in at the door, and filled the lower story of the house. They had nowhere to remove their household goods, and stored them in the garret carefully packed, and went out to find a shelter in an old log house near by, used for a corn-crib. Day by day they watched the house, hailed passing boats for news of the rise and fall of the water above, always trusting the house would stand—" and it would," the mother said, " for it was a good, strong house, but for the storm." The winds came, and the terrible gale that swept the valley like a tornado, with the water at its height, leveling whole towns, descended and beat upon that house, and it fell. In the morning there was no house there, and the waves in their fury rushed madly on. Then these little children " stood and wept on the banks of the river," and the desolation and fear in the careful mother's heart, none but herself and her God can know.

They lived on in the corn-crib, and it was from it they came to hail us as we passed to-day. Something had been told us of them on our downward trip, and a package had been left them at " Cave-in Rock," which they had not received. We went over shoe-tops in mud to their rude home, to find it one room of logs, an old stone chimney, with a cheerful fire of drift-wood and a *clean* hearth, two wrecks of beds, a table, and two chairs which some kind neighbor had loaned. The Government boats had left them rations. There was an air of thrift, even in their desolation, a plank walk was laid about the door, the floor was cleanly swept, and . the twenty-five surviving hens, for an equal number were lost in the storm, clucked and craiked comfortably about the door, and there were two-and-a-half dozen fresh eggs to sell us at a higher rate than paid in town. We stood, as we had done so many scores of times during the last few weeks, and looked this pitiful scene in the face. There were misfortune, poverty, sorrow, want, loneliness, dread of the future, but fortitude, courage, integrity, and honest thrift.

"Would she like to return to the childhood home in Indiana?" we asked the mother, for we would help them go.

"No," she said tenderly. "My husband lived and died here. He is buried here, and I would not like to go away and leave him alone. It won't be very long, and it is a comfort to the children to be able to visit his grave. No, I reckon we will stay here, and out of the wreck of the old house which sticks up out of the mud, we will put up another

little hut, higher up on the bank out of the way
of the floods, and if it is only a hut, it will be a
home for us and we will get into it, and make our
crop this year."

There were no dry eyes, but very still hearts,
while we listened to this sorrowful but brave little
speech, made with a voice full of tears.

Our thoughtful field agent, Dr. Hubbell, was the
first to speak.

" Here are six children," he said with an inquir-
ing glance at me.

No response was needed. The thing was done.
We told the mother the story of " The Little Six "
of Waterford, and asked her if that money with
enough more to make up one hundred dollars would
help her to get up her house? It was *her* turn to
be speechless. At length with a struggling, choking voice she managed to say—"God knows how
much it would be to me. Yes, with my good boys
I can do it, and do it well."

We put in her hands a check for this sum, and
directed from the boat clean boxes of clothing and
bedding, to help restore the household, when the
house should have been completed.

Before we left her, we asked if she would name

her house when it should be done? She thought a second, and caught the idea.

" Yes," she replied quickly, with a really winsome smile on that worn and weary face, " yes, I shall name it ' The Little Six.' "

We came to Pittsburg, discharged our empty boat, bade a heart-breaking good-by to our veteran volunteers from Evansville, who had shared our toil and pain and who would return on the boat, we taking train once more for Washington. We had been four months on the rivers, among fogs, rain, damp, and malaria—run all manner of risks and dangers, but had lost no life nor property, sunk no boat, and only that I was by this time too weak to walk without help—all were well.

Through the thoughtfulness of our new societies—St. Louis and Chicago—we had been able to meet our share of the expenses, and to keep good the little personal provision we started with, and were thus ready to commence another field when it should come.

On arriving home I found that I was notified by the International Committee of Geneva, that the Fourth International Conference would be held in that city in September, and I was requested to inform the United States Government, and ask it to send delegates. With the aid of a borrowed arm, I made my way up the steps of the Department of State (that was before the luxury of elevators) and made my errand known to Secretary Frelinghuysen, who had heard of it and was ready with his reply:

"Yes, Miss Barton, we will make the needful appointment of delegates to the International Conference, and I appoint you as our delegate."

"No, Mr. Frelinghuysen," I said, "I can not go. I have just returned from field work. I am tired and ill. Furthermore, I have not had time to make a report of our work."

"There is no one else who sufficiently understands the Red Cross, and the provisions of the treaty, that our Government can send, and we can not afford to make a mistake in the matter of delegates to this first conference in which our Government shall participate," answered the Secretary. "As to the report, have you not acknowledged the contributions to all those who have sent?"

"Oh, yes; every dollar and every box of goods where the donor was known," I replied.

28

" Has any one complained? " he asked.

" No; not a single person so far as is known. We have had only thanks."

" Then to whom would you report? "

" To you, Mr. Secretary, or to such person or in such manner as you shall designate."

" I don't want any report; no report is necessary," answered the Secretary. " Our Government relief-boats have reported you officially, and all the country knows what you have done and is more than satisfied. Regarding your illness—you have had too much fresh water, Miss Barton, I recommend salt—and shall appoint you."

This was done, and the appropriation for expenses was made, and at my request Judge Joseph Sheldon, and by invitation Mr. A. S. Solomon, our vice-president, were also appointed to accompany me. The appropriation sufficed for all.

The conference was held at Geneva, September 17, 1884, and thus was had the first official representation of the United States Government at an International Conference of the Treaty of Geneva. There have since been five. I have attended all but one.

II

BEFORE the close of the following year, 1885, came what was known as the " Texas Famine." Thousands of miles of wild land, forming the Pan Handle, had been suddenly opened by the building of a Southern Railroad. In the speculative anxiety of the Road to people its newly acquired territory, unwarranted inducements of climatic advantages had been unscrupulously held out to the poor farmers of Mississippi, Alabama, and Georgia.

Lured by the pictures presented them, some thousands of families had been induced to leave their old, worn-out farms, and with the little they could carry or drive, reach the new Eldorado, to find a new farm that needed only the planting to make them rich, prosperous, and happy, without labor. They planted. The first year brought some returns—the second was a drought with no returns—the third the same. Hunger for them-

selves and starvation for their stock stared them
in the face. They could not pick up and go back
—the rivers were dry from the Rio Grande to the
Brazos—the earth was iron, and the heavens brass;
cattle wandered at will for water and feed, and
their bones whitened the plains.

These were poor little peoples. They tried to
make the great State know of their distress, but
the rich railroad proprietors held the *press*, and no
one knew their condition or could get correct information. At length a faithful clergyman came
to Washington, to President Cleveland, and the
Red Cross.

We consulted with the President, who gave encouragement for us to go to Texas and learn the
facts.

In mid-winter, 1886, accompanied by Dr. Hubbell, the journey was undertaken. We proceeded
to Albany, Texas, made headquarters—traveled
over the stricken counties, found wretchedness,
hunger, thirst, cold, heart-breaking discourage-
ment. The third year of drought was upon them,
and the good people of that great State, misled
by its press, its press in turn misled by the specu-

lators, innocently discredited every report of distress, and amused themselves by little sly innuendoes and witty jokes on the " Texas Famine."

The condition was pitiful. To them it was hopeless. And yet not a dollar or a pound was needed outside of Texas. They only required to know the truth. This then was our task. We ceased to journey over arid fields of suffering, and turned our steps resolutely to the editorial rooms of the Dallas and Galveston News, at Dallas. Both editors were present; both sat half-breathless while the flood of information rolled over them in no uncertain terms.

I shall never forget the tears in the mild blue eyes of General Belo, as he learned what he had done, and was still doing. Twelve hours brought another issue of the two papers. A column of editorial told the true situation. A modest contribution of the Red Cross headed a subscription list, General Belo following with his, and almost immediately the legislature made an appropriation of one hundred thousand dollars for food and supplies.

The tender-hearted and conscience-smitten people sent their donations. Our task was done. We had seen and conquered.

In the midst of a cold rain in February we reached Washington. A concise and full report was made to President Cleveland, saying in conclusion: "I thank you with all my heart, Mr. President, for the encouragement at the commencement, and for the privilege of writing you. We have done this little bit of work faithfully and hope it may meet your approval."

President Cleveland's letter of thanks still bears testimony of his care for the people of the country, and his faith in its institutions.

Not a dollar of outside help passed through our hands, but the little permanent provision was equal to the occasion and we had still a half left of our three thousand dollars. That was our first acquaintance with Texas. Galveston followed many years later with the same firm accord and good results. The bonds of affection had grown deep and strong between the great thousand-mile State and the little Red Cross that loved to serve her.

In the following year, 1887, we were notified by the International Committee of Geneva of the con-

ference to be held at Carlsruhe, by invitation of
the Grand Duke and Grand Duchess of Baden.
We were directed to inform the Department of
State of this fact. We did so, and an appropriation was made by Congress to defray the expenses
of three delegates.

It may be well to explain that in these appoint-
ments the Government does not place the appropriation in the hands of the appointees, but simply
becomes a guaranty. The appointee provides his
own funds. If, after return, vouchers can be
shown that the sum guaranteed has been spent according to regulations, he is reimbursed in due
course.

Here was at least a contrast from a rough Mississippi River boat and the crude homes of an un-
settled Western State, to the royal carriage waiting to convey one to the apartments reserved in a
palace, the elegance and culture of a court, the
precision of a congress of representatives of the
nations of the world. The questions of humanity
discussed by them, the meeting of friends of other
days, the regal bearing of the royal host and
hostess, the last parting from the dear old Em-

peror of ninety-two, and his tenderly spoken, " It is the last time, good-by "; the loving and last farewell of the beloved Empress Augusta, the patron saint of the Red Cross; Bismarck and Moltke, in review, each with his Red Cross insignia; the cordial hand grasp and the farewell never repeated—and all of this attention to and interest in a subject that the country I had gone to represent scarcely realized had an existence beyond the receiving of some second-hand clothing, misfit shoes, and a little money sent by some one to some place, where something bad had happened.

No one dreamed that it meant anything more, or that it needed anything after this, and nothing more was done.

It is only now, after almost two decades and within the last three months, that we commence to awaken and wonder, with a mingled national and personal sense of indignation, why our American Red Cross is not as rich and great as in other nations?

In February, 1888, occurred the Mt. Vernon, Ill., cyclone, cutting a broad swath through one-half of the beautiful county-seat, tearing down all heavy buildings, picking up the lighter ones and sweeping them along like cardboard.

In three minutes the work of destruction was over. Ten minutes later the sun shone out brightly over the ruins of the town, the wails of the maimed and dying, and the lifeless bodies of the dead.

Fires broke out on every hand, and the victims pinned down under the wreckage were subjects for the flames. Appeals for assistance went out, but by unfortunate press representation failed to arouse the public, till after several days, when we were reached, through their representative in Congress, begging that in mercy we go to them. We arrived in the night, found homes destroyed, hospitals full, scant medical care, few nurses, food scarce and no money, a relief committee of excellent men, but little to distribute.

At daylight we looked over the situation and sent this simple message to the Associated Press:

" The pitiless snow is falling on the heads of three thousand people, who are without homes, without food or clothing, and without money.

" AMERICAN NATIONAL RED CROSS,

" Clara Barton, President."

This was all. We assisted their relief committee to arrange for the receipt and distribution of funds, sent for experienced helpers to take charge of supplies, to distribute clothing, and aid the hospital service. We remained two weeks, and left them with more supplies than they knew how to distribute, and the Citizens' Committee, with accumulating cash in its treasury of ninety thousand dollars, full of hope, life, and a gratitude they could not speak.

As in the Texas famine, we paid our own expenses and no dollar but our own had passed our hands. We were only glad to do this, in the hope that we were building up an institution of self-help of the people, that would one day win its way to their favor and aid.

III

DURING the same year the yellow fever broke out in Jacksonville, Fla., and was declared epidemic in September.

An arrangement had been made between the National Association and the Auxiliary Society of the Red Cross of New Orleans, which society embraced the famous old " Howard Association," that, in case of an outbreak of yellow fever, they would send their immune nurses from the South, and we of the North would supply the money to support and pay them.

This arrangement was carried out so far as could be, under the very natural differences of a medical department of active, professional men, taking up the treatment of an epidemic of which they knew very little experimentally, but filled with the enthusiasm of science and hope, and the unprofessional, fearless, easy-going gait of the old Southern nurses, white and black, whose whole lives had been spent in just that work.

38

The Red Cross sent no Northern nurses. But eighteen or twenty " Howard nurses," mainly colored, went out from New Orleans under charge of Col. Fred. F. Southmayd, their leader of twenty years in epidemics. A part of his nurses were stationed at Macclenny, and a part went on to Jacksonville. Under medical direction of their noted " yellow fever doctor "—a tall Norwegian— Dr. Gill, they did their faithful work and won their meed of grateful praise.

Our place was in Washington, to receive, deal carefully with, and hold back the tide of offered service from the hundreds of enthusiastic, excited untrained volunteers, rushing on to danger and death. Their fearless ignorance was a pitiful lesson. In all the hundreds there was scarcely one who had ever seen a case of yellow fever, but all were sure they were proof against it. Only three passed us, and two of these had the fever in Jacksonville.

When the scourge was ended we met our nurses personally at Camp Perry, paid and sent them back to New Orleans. All that are living are at our service still, faithful and true.

During the fourth week in November a dispatch
to national headquarters announced that the last
band of Red Cross nurses, known as the " Macclenny Nurses," had finished their work at Enterprise, and would come into Camp Perry to wait
their ten days' quarantine and go home to New
Orleans for Thanksgiving.

That would mean that seventy-nine days ago
their little company of eighteen, mainly women,
steaming on to Jacksonville, under guidance of
their old-time trusted leader, Southmayd, of New
Orleans, listened to his announcement that the town
of Macclenny, thirty-eight miles from Jacksonville, Fla., and through which they would soon pass,
was in a fearful state of distress; a comparatively
new town, of a few thousand, largely Northern and
Western people, suddenly stricken down in scores;
poor, helpless, physicians all ill, and no nurses;
quarantined on all sides, no food, medicine, nor
comforts for sick or well.

" Nurses, shall I leave a part of you there; the
train can not stop in, nor near the town, but if I
can manage to get it slowed up somewhere, will
you jump? "

"We will do anything you say, colonel; we are here in God's name and service to help His people; for Him, for you, and for the Red Cross, we will do our best and our all."

"Conductor, you had a hot box a few miles back; don't you think it should be looked to after passing Macclenny?"

"I will slow up and have it seen to, colonel, although it may cost me my official head." And it did.

One mile beyond town, the rain pouring in torrents, the ground soaked, slippery, and caving, out into pitchy darkness, leaped three men and seven women from a puffing, unsteady train, no physician with them, and no instructions save the charge of their leader as the last leap was made, and the train pushed on: "Nurses, you know what to do; go and do your best, and God help you." Hand to hand, that none go astray in the darkness, they hobbled back over a mile of slippery cross-ties to the stricken town. Shelter was found, the wet clothes dried, and at midnight the sick had been parceled out, each nurse had his or her quota of patients, and were in for the issue, be it life or

4   41

death. Those past all help must be seen through, and lost, all that could be must be saved. The next day a dispatch from Southmayd went back to New Orleans for Dr. Gill to come and take charge of the sick and the nurses at Macclenny. It was done, and under his wise direction they found again a leader. Their labors and successes are matters for later and more extended record.

It is to be borne in mind that these nurses found no general table, no table at all but such as they could provide, find the food for, and cook for themselves, for the sick, the children, and the old and helpless who had escaped the fever and must be cared for. No patient could be left till the crisis was passed, and many are their records of seventy-two hours without change or sleep or scarcely sitting down. As the disease gradually succumbed to their watchful care, experience, and skill, they reached out to other freshly attacked towns and hamlets. Sanderson and Glen St. Mary's became their charge, and return their blessings for lives preserved.

On November 1st it was thought they could safely leave and go into camp for quarantine; but no regular train would be permitted to take them. The Red Cross secured and paid a special train for them, and, as if in bold relief against the manner of their entry seven weeks before, the entire town, saving its invalids, was assembled at the station at seven o'clock in the morning to bid them good-by and God speed.

But their fame had gone before them, and " Enterprise," a hundred miles below, just stricken down among its flowers and fruits, reached out its hands for aid, and with one accord, after two days in camp, all turned back from the coveted home and needed rest and added another month of toil to their already weary record. At length this was ended, and word came again to us that they would go into quarantine. Their unselfish, faithful, and successful record demanded something more than the mere sending of money. It deserved the thanks of the Red Cross organization in the best and highest manner in which they could be bestowed; it was decided that its President, in person, should most fittingly do this, and I accordingly left Washington on the morning of November 22d in company with Dr. Hubbell, field agent, for Camp

43

Perry, the quarantine station of Florida. Two days and one night by rail, a few miles across country by wagon, where trains were forbidden to stop, and another mile or so over the trestles of St. Mary's on a dirt car with the workmen, brought us into camp as the evening fires were lighted and the bugle sounded supper. The genial surgeon in charge, Dr. Hutton, who carried a knapsack and musket in an Illinois regiment in '62, met us cordially and extended every possible hospitality. Soon there filed past us to supper the tall doctor and his little flock; some light and fair-skinned, with the easy step of a well-bred lady, others dark and bony-handed, but the strong, kind faces below the turbans told at a glance that you could trust your life there and find it again. They were not disturbed that night, and no certain information of our arrival got among them. It was cold and windy, and the evening short, as nine o'clock brought taps and lights out. In spite of all caution the news of our coming had spread over the surrounding country, and telegrams bringing both thanks for what had been received and the needs for more, came from all sides, and the good Mayor of Macclenny made his troubled way to reach and greet us in person, and take again the faithful hands that had served and saved his people.

Surgeon Hutton's headquarter tent was politely tendered for the first meeting, and as one could never, while memory lasts, forget this scene, so no words can ever adequately describe it. The ample tent was filled. Here on the right the Mayor, broad shouldered, kind faced and efficient, officers of camp, and many visitors, wondering what it all meant; in the center the tall doctor and his faithful band—Eliza Lanier, Lena Seymour (mother and daughter), Elizabeth Eastman, Harriet Schmidt, Lizzie Louis, Rebecca Vidal, Annie Evans, Arthur Duteil, Frederick Wilson, and Edward Holyland.

I give these names because they are worthy a place in the history of any epidemic; but no country, race, nor creed could claim them as a body: four Americans, one German, one French, one Irish, three Africans, part Protestant, and part Catholic, but all from New Orleans, of grand old *Howard* stock, from Memphis down, nursing in every epidemic from the bayous of the Mississippi

45

to Tampa Bay; and hereafter we will know them
as the "*Old Guard.*"

Here, in the winds of approaching winter they
stand in the light garb of early September in New
Orleans, thin, worn, longing for home, but patient,
grateful, and glad, some trifling "nubia" or
turban about the head, but only one distinguishing
feature in common. A pitiful little misshapen Red
Cross, made by their own hands, of two bits of
scarlet ribbon, soiled, fringed, and tattered, pinned
closely upon the left breast of each, strove in mute
appeal to say who they were, and what they served.
A friendly recognition and some words of thanks
from their President, opened the way for those
anxious to follow. The rich, warm eloquence of
Mayor Watkins plainly told from how near his
heart the stream of gratitude was flowing, and his
manly voice trembled as he reverted to the condition of his stricken people, on that pitiless night,
when this little band of pilgrim strangers strayed
back to them in the rain and darkness. "I fear
they often worked in hunger," he said, "for then,
as now, we had little for ourselves, our sick, or our
well; but they brought us to our feet, and the bless-

46

ing of every man, woman, and child in Macclenny is on them."

It was with a kind of paternal pride that Dr. Gill advanced and placed before us his matchless record of cases attended, and life preserved. " This is the record of our work," he said. " I am proud of it, and glad that I have been able to make it, but without the best efforts of these faithful nurses I could not have done it; they have stood firm through everything; not a word of complaint from, nor of, one of them, in all these trying months, and I thank you, our President, for this opportunity to testify to their merits in your presence." The full cups overflowed, and as we took each brown calloused hand in ours, and felt the warm tears dropping over them, we realized how far from calloused were the hearts behind them. The silence that followed was a season of prayer.

Then came opportunity for some conversation, questions, and explanations. " We wish to introduce to our President our chief nurse, whom Colonel Southmayd placed in charge of us when we left the car, and directed us to obey him; he is younger than any of us, Ed. Holyland." A slight young

man with clear, olive complexion, and dark-browed
earnest eyes that looked you straight in the face,
came forward; his apparent youthfulness gave rise
to the first remark:

"How old are you, Mr. Holyland?"

"Twenty-nine, madam."

"And you have taken charge of these nurses?"

"I have done what I could for their comfort; I
think that was what the colonel desired; he knew
they would need only care and advice, they would
do their best of themselves. During the few days
that Colonel Southmayd remained in Jacksonville,"
he continued, "he was able to send us some such
comforts as we needed for the sick, and some nour-
ishing food for ourselves; but this was only a few
days, you know, and after that we got on as well
as we could without. I know that after he left the
nurses gave to the sick, the children, the old and
the helpless, what they needed for their own
strength."

"But you did not tell us this, Mr. Holyland."

"No, we were dazed and frightened by the
things we heard. We felt that your organization
was having enough to bear. We knew we must

look to you for our pay, and we thought, under the circumstances, that would be your share. But permit me, please, to call your attention to Mr. Wilson (a stout colored man advanced), who took charge of a little hospital of six cases, and carried them all through, day and night, without an hour's relief from any person, and never lost a single case."

"And permit me," chimed in the clear-toned Irish voice of Lizzie Louis, "to tell of Mr. Holyland himself, who found a neglected Italian family a mile or more outside of the town. He went and nursed them alone, and when the young son, a lad of thirteen or fourteen years, died, knowing there was no one to bury him there, he wrapped him in a blanket and brought him into town on his back, for burial."

Holyland's face grew sad, and his eyes modestly sought the floor, as he listened to this unexpected revelation.

"I wish to speak of something else," added one of the men, "which we were held back from doing, and for which we are now very glad. We should not have thought of it ourselves. It is cus-

49

tomary," he continued, " when a patient dies in an epidemic, to give the nurse ten dollars for preparing the body for burial; this was done in our first case, but Mr. Holyland had the gift promptly returned with thanks, and the explanation that we were employed by an organization which fully rewarded its nurses, and was too high and too correct to accept tribute for misfortune; it was enough that the patient was lost."

By this time poor black Annie Evans, the " Mammy " of the group, could hold quiet no longer, and broke silence with, " Missus President! whar is de colonel? Colonel Southmayd; dey tells me all de time he's gone away from New Orleans, and I can't b'l'eve 'em. He can't go away; he can't lib anywhar else, he was always dar. I'se nursed in yellow fever and cholera more'n twenty-five year, and I neber went for nobody but him; it arn't no New Orleans for us widout him dar. I doesn't know de name of dat place dey say he's gone to, and I doesn't want to; he'll be in New Orleans when we gets dar."

There were pitying glances among the group, at this little burst of feeling, for in some way it was an echo of their own; and Lena Seymour added tenderly: "We have been trying for these two months to convince Mammy about this, but she is firm in her faith and sometimes refuses to hear us." But the subject changed with "How many cases did you lose in this epidemic, Mammy?"

"I didn't lose no cases! Lor' bless you, honey, I doesn't lose cases if dey hasn't been killed afore dey gets to me; folks needn't die of yellow fever."

We didn't suppose that "Mammy" intended any reflection upon the medical fraternity.

"But now, friends, we must turn to our settlement, which can not be difficult. Three dollars a day for each nurse, for seventy-nine days, till you are home on Thanksgiving morning. But here are only ten. There are eighteen on our list who left with you and Colonel Southmayd; where are your comrades?" Some eyes flashed and some moistened, as they answered, "We do not know." "They remained in the car that night, and went on to Jacksonville." Swift, dark glances swept from one to another among them. Instinctively they drew closer to each other, and over knitted brows and firmly set teeth, a silence fell dark and

51

ominous like a pall, which the future alone can lift.

The bugle sounded dinner, and this ended our little camp-meeting, than which few camp-meetings, we believe, ever came nearer to the heart of Him who offered His life a ransom, and went about doing good.

The winds blew cold across the camp; the fires shot out long angry tongues of flame and drifts of smoke to every passer-by. The norther was upon us. Night came down, and all were glad of shelter and sleep. The morning, quiet, crisp, and white with frost, revealed the blessing which had fallen upon a stricken land.

Thanksgiving was there before its time. The hard rules relaxed. One day more, and the quarantine was at an end. The north-bound train halted below the camp, and all together, President and agent, tall doctor and happy nurses, took places on it, the first for headquarters at Washington, the last for New Orleans, and home for Thanksgiving morning, full of the joys of a duty well done, rich in well-paid labor, in the love of those they had befriended, and the approval of a whole people, South and North, when once their work should be known to them.

To the last, they clung to their little home-made Red Crosses as if they had been gold and diamonds; and when at length the tracks diverged and the parting must be made, it was with few words, low and softly spoken, but meaning much, with a finger touch upon the little cross, " When you want us, we are there."

The supplies forwarded by us were estimated at ten thousand dollars. The money received was $6,281.58. Out of this sum we paid our twenty nurses three dollars a day, for seventy-nine days—their cost of living, and their transportation when needed. We paid our doctor in charge twenty dollars a day, the customary price, for the same period. We paid our office rent, assistants, telegraphing, drayage for supplies sent on by us (railroad transportation free), and all incidentals for a relief work of over three months' duration. This ran our debit column over on the other side over one thousand dollars. Our little part of the relief of that misfortune was estimated at fifteen thousand dollars, and only those relieved were more grateful than we.   53

IV

On Sunday afternoon, May 31, 1889, with the waters of the Potomac two feet deep on Pennsylvania Avenue, a half dozen of us left Washington for Johnstown, over washed-out ties and broken tracks, with every little gully swollen to a raging torrent. After forty-eight hours of this, we reached the scene, which no one need or could describe, but if ever a people needed help it was these.

Scarcely a house standing that was safe to enter, the wrecks piled in rubbish thirty feet in height, four thousand dead in the river beds, twenty thousand foodless but for Pittsburg bread rations, and a cold rain which continued unbroken by sunshine for forty days.

It was at the moment of supreme affliction when we arrived at Johnstown. The waters had subsided, and those of the inhabitants who had escaped the fate of their fellows were gazing over the scene

54

of destruction and trying to arouse themselves from the lethargy that had taken hold of them when they were stunned by the realization of all the woe that had been visited upon them. How nobly they responded to the call of duty! How much of the heroic there is in our people when it is needed! No idle murmurings of fate, but true to the god-like instincts of manhood and fraternal love, they quickly banded together to do the best that the wisest among them could suggest.

For five weary months it was our portion to live amid the scenes of destruction, desolation, poverty, want and woe; sometimes in tents, sometimes without; and so much rain and mud, and such a lack of the commonest comforts for a time, until we could build houses to shelter ourselves and those around us. Without a safe and with a dry-goods box for a desk, we conducted financial affairs in money and material to the extent of nearly half a million dollars.

I shall never lose the memory of my first walk on the first day—the wading in mud, the climbing over broken engines, cars, heaps of iron rollers, broken timbers, wrecks of houses; bent railway tracks tangled with piles of iron wire; bands of workmen, squads of military, and getting around the bodies of dead animals, and often people being borne away; the smouldering fires and drizzling rain—all for the purpose of officially announcing to the commanding general (for the place was under martial law) that the Red Cross had arrived in the field. I could not have puzzled General Hastings more if I had addressed him in Chinese; and if ours had been truly an Oriental mission, the gallant soldier could not have been more courteous and kind. He immediately set about devising means for making as comfortable as possible a " poor, lone woman," helpless, of course, upon such a field. It was with considerable difficulty that I could convince him that the Red Cross had a way of taking care of itself at least, and was not likely to suffer from neglect.

Not a business house or bank left, the safes all in the bottom of the river; our little pocketbook was useless, there was nothing to buy, and it would not bring back the dead. With the shelter of the tents of the Philadelphia Red Cross, that joined us en route with supplies, when we could find a cleared place to spread, or soil to hold them, with a dry-goods box for a desk, our stenographer commenced to rescue the first dispatches of any description that entered that desolate city. The disturbed rivers lapped wearily back and forth, the people, dazed and dumb, dug in the muddy banks for their dead. Hastings with his little army of militia kept order.

Soon supplies commenced to pour in from every-where, to be received, sheltered as best they could be from the incessant rain, and distributed by hu-man hands, for it was three weeks before even a cart could pass the streets.

But I am not here to describe Johnstown—the noble help that came to it, nor the still more noble people that received it—but simply to say that the little untried and unskilled Red Cross played its minor tune of a single fife among the grand chorus of relief of the whole country, that rose like an anthem, till over four millions in money, contrib-uted to its main body of relief, with the faithful Kreamer at its head, had modestly taken the place of the twelve millions destroyed. But after all it was largely the supplies that saved the people at first, as it always is, and the distribution of which largely consumed the money that was contributed later.

From one mammoth tent which served as a warehouse, food and clothing were given out to the waiting people through the hands of such volunteer agents, both women and men, as I scarcely dare hope to ever see gathered together in one work again. The great cry which had gone out had aroused the entire country, and our old-time helpers, full of rich experience and still richer love for the work, faithful to the cross of humanity as the devotee to the cross of the Master, came up from every point—the floods, the cyclones; the battlefields—and kneeling before the shrine, pledged heart and service anew to the work. Fair hands laying aside their diamonds, and business men their cares, left homes of elegance and luxury to open rough boxes and barrels, handle second-hand clothing, eat coarse food at rough-board tables, sleep on cots under a dripping canvas tent, all for the love of humanity symbolized in the little flag that floated above them.

Clergymen left their pulpits and laymen their charge to tramp over the hillsides from house to house, to find who needed and suffered, and to carry to them from our tents on their shoulders, like beasts of burden, the huge bundles of relief, where no beast of burden could reach.

We had been early requested by official resolution of the Finance Committee of the City of Johnstown to aid them in the erection of houses. We accepted the invitation, and at the same time proposed to aid in furnishing the nucleus of a household for the home which should in any way be made up. This aid seemed imperative, as nothing was left for them to commence living with, neither beds, chairs, tables, nor cooking utensils of any kind; and there were few if any stores open, and no furniture in town.

Of this labor we had our share. Six buildings of one hundred feet by fifty, later known as " Red Cross Hotels," were quickly put up to shelter the people, furnished, supplied, and kept like hotels, free of all cost to them, while others were built by the general committee. Three thousand of the latter were erected, and the Red Cross furnished every one with substantial, newly purchased furniture, ready for occupancy. The books of the

"Titusville Manufacturing Company" will show one cash order of ten thousand dollars for furniture. The three thousand houses thus furnished each accommodated two families.

A ponderous book of nearly two feet square shows the name, sex, and number of persons of each family, and a list of every article received by them. To-day one looks in wonder at such a display of clerical labor and accuracy, under even favorable conditions.

This was only accomplished by the hard, unpaid labor of every officer, and the large amount of volunteer friendly aid that came to us.

The great manufacturers of the country, and the heavy contributing agents, on learning our intentions, sent, without a hint from us, many of their articles, as, for instance, New Bedford, Mass., sent mattresses and bedding; Sheboygan, Wis., sent furniture and enameled ironware; Titusville, Pa., with a population of ten thousand, sent ten thousand dollars' worth of its well-made bedsteads, springs, extension-tables, chairs, stands and rockers; and the well-known New York newspaper, The Mail and Express, sent a large lot of mattresses, feather pillows, bedclothing, sheets, and pillow-slips by the thousand and cooking utensils by the ten thousands. Six large teams were in constant service delivering these goods.

When the contributions slackened or ceased, and more material was needed, we purchased of the same firms which had contributed, keeping our stock good until all applications were filled. The record on our books showed that over twenty-five thousand persons had been directly served by us. They had received our help independently and — without begging. No child has learned to beg at the doors of the Red Cross.

It is to be borne in mind that the fury of the deluge had swept almost entirely the homes of the wealthy, the elegant, the cultured leaders of society, and the fathers of the town. This class who were spared were more painfully homeless than the indigent poor, who could still huddle in together. They could not go away, for the suffering and demoralized town needed their care and oversight more than ever before. There was no home for them, nowhere to get a meal of food or to sleep. Still they must work on, and the stranger coming

61

to town on business must go unfed, with no shelter
at night, if he would sleep, or, indeed, escape being
picked up by the military guard.

To meet these necessities, and being apprehen-
sive that some good lives might go out under the
existing lack of accommodations, it was decided to
erect a building similar to our warehouse. The
use of the former site of the Episcopal Church was
generously tendered us by the Bishop early in
June, for any purpose we might desire. This
house, which was soon erected, was known as the
" Locust Street Red Cross Hotel"; it stood some
fifty rods from our warehouse, and was fifty by one
hundred and sixteen feet in dimensions, two stories
in height, with lantern roof, built of hemlock, single siding, papered inside with heavy building
paper, and heated by natural gas, as all our buildings were. It consisted of thirty-four rooms, besides kitchen, laundry, bath-rooms with hot and
cold water, and one main dining-hall and sitting-
room through the center, sixteen feet in width by
one hundred in length.

It was fully furnished with excellent beds, bedding, bureaus, tables, chairs, and all needful house-

keeping furniture. A competent landlady, who, like the rest, had a few weeks before floated down over the same ground on the roof of her house in thirty feet of water, was placed in charge, with instructions to keep a good house, make what she could rent free, but charging no Johnstown person over twenty-five cents for a meal of food.

This was the first attempt at social life after that terrible separation, and its success was something that I am very proud of. The house was full of townspeople from the first day, and strangers no longer looked in vain for accommodations.

The conception of the need of this house, and the method of selecting its inmates, and the manner of inducting them into their new home, were somewhat unique and may be of interest to the reader. I had noticed among the brave and true men, who were working in the mud and rain, many refined-looking gentlemen, who were, before this great misfortune carried away most of their belongings, the wealthiest and most influential citizens. Never having had to struggle amid such hardships and deprivations, their sufferings were more acute than those of the poorer and more

hardy people; and it did not require any great
foresight to know that they were physically in-
capable of such labor if prolonged, nor to predict
their early sickness and death if they were not properly housed and fed. As the salvation of the town
depended in a great measure upon the efforts of
these men, it was vitally necessary that their lives
should be preserved. Realizing all this, it occurred
to us that the most important thing to do, next to
feeding the hungry, was to provide proper shelter
for these delicate men and their families. The
idea once conceived was soon communicated to my
staff, and, after due consideration, it was put in
the way of realization.

On the afternoon of July 27th hundreds of citizens called on us, and congratulations and good
wishes were the order of the day. As the members
of each family whom we had selected to occupy
apartments in the house arrived, they were quietly
taken aside and requested to remain and have dinner with us. After all the guests were departed
except those who had been requested to remain,
dinner was announced, and the party was seated by
the members of the Red Cross. Beside the plate

of each head of a family were laid the keys to an apartment, with a card inviting the family to take possession at once, and remain as long as they chose.

I can not describe the scene that followed; there were tears and broken voices; suffice to say, the members of that household were made happy and comfortable for many long months; and I venture to assert that those now living recall those days with the fondest recollections.

The contributions to the general committee had been so liberal that it was possible to erect and provide for the great burial-place of its dead— "Grand View," that overlooks the city. It was also suggested that a benevolent society, as a permanent institution, be formed by the united action of the general committee and the Red Cross. This was successfully accomplished by the generous provision of eight thousand dollars from the committee on its part and the turning over of our well-made and supplied hospital buildings, and the funds we had left placed in charge of a faithful custodian under our pay for the following six months.

This is the present "Union Benevolent Society" of Johnstown to-day.

I remained five months with these people without once visiting my own home, only returning to it when the frost had killed the green I had left in May.

In that time, it was estimated, we had housed, handled, and distributed $211,000 worth of supplies—new and old—for, by request of the weary chairman of the general committee, at the last, we took up the close of its distribution. It is our joy and pride to recall how closely we worked in connection with that honored committee from first to last, and how strong and unsullied that friendship has remained.

The value of money that passed through our hands was $39,000, as stated in the official report of the general committee, to which all required returns were made, recorded, and published by the committee.

Our usual quota of assistants was fifty persons, the higher grade of men and women assistants largely volunteers. Two railroads brought our supplies. To handle these the strongest men were required, and seven two-horse teams ran daily for three and a half months in the distribution, at customary rates of pay. These were the workingmen of the town who had suffered with the rest.

It was a joy that in all the uncertainties of that uncertain field not a single complaint ever reached us of the non-acknowledgment of a dollar entrusted to us.

The paths of charity are over roadways of ashes; and he who would tread them must be prepared to meet opposition, misconstruction, jealousy, and calumny. Let his work be that of angels —still it will not satisfy all.

In the light of recent events, I may perhaps be pardoned for quoting a few lines from the official report of the Johnstown Flood Finance Committee appointed by Governor Beaver, as showing how these gentlemen, the foremost men in the community, regarded our efforts to give them a helping hand:

" In this matter of sheltering the people, as in others of like importance, Miss Clara Barton, President of the Red Cross Association, was most helpful. At a time when there was a doubt if the

Flood Commission could furnish houses of suitable
character and with the requisite promptness, she
offered to assume charge, and she erected with the
funds of the Association three large apartment
houses, which afforded comfortable lodgings for
many houseless people. She was among the first
to arrive on the scene of calamity, bringing with
her Dr. Hubbell, the Field Officer of the Red Cross
Association, and a staff of skilled assistants. She
made her own organization for relief work in every
form, disposing of the large resources under her
control with such wisdom and tenderness that the
charity of the Red Cross had no sting, and its re-
cipients are not Miss Barton's dependents, but her
friends. She was also the last of the ministering
spirits to leave the scene of her labors, and she left
her apartment houses for use during the winter,
and turned over her warehouse with its store of
furniture, bedding, and clothing, and a well-
equipped infirmary, to the Union Benevolent Association of the Conemaugh Valley, the organization
of which she advised and helped to form; and its
lady visitors have so well performed their work that
the dreaded winter has no terrors, mendicancy has

68

been repressed, and not a single case of unrelieved suffering is known to have occurred in all the flooded district."

Enterprising, industrious, and hopeful, the new Johnstown, phœnix-like, rose from its ruins more beautiful than the old, with a ceaseless throb of grateful memory for every kind act rendered, and every thought of sympathy given her in her great hour of desolation and woe. God bless her, and God bless all who helped save her!

V

As early as 1889, the foreign journals began to tell us of the apprehension caused by an unusual failure, of the crops in Central Russia, extending from Moscow north and south, and east beyond the Ural Mountains and into Siberia—embracing an era of a million square miles. This failure was followed by another in 1890.

Eighteen hundred and ninety-one found the old-time granaries empty, and a total failure of the crops, and a population of thirty-five millions of people, paralyzed with the dread of approaching famine.

The American Red Cross had placed itself in communication with the Secretary of State, Hon. James G. Blaine, whose name and memory it treasures with reverence, and Mr. Alexander Gregor, the accomplished Russian *Chargé d'Affaires* at Washington, and ascertained that Russia would gladly receive donations of relief from

America. She would even send her ships for any food that might be offered. This, America would not permit and Congress was appealed to for ocean transportation. The Senate voted a liberal appropriation, which was defeated in the House.

Then the Red Cross, with the aid of the citizens of Washington, took up the matter. They were joined by the Order of Elks, which contributed a sum of seven hundred dollars, than which perhaps that liberal Order never made a more timely gift. Funds were raised to charter a steamship for the Red Cross. The spirit spread generally over the country. Philadelphia sent a messenger to learn what Washington was doing, and was advised to charter one of its own ships, which was done, and two consignments were finally made by them.

Minnesota had already acted, and later, by the advice and aid of the extra provision of the Red Cross, the Christian Herald sent out its ship cargo, under convoy of Rev. Dr. Talmage.

But the State of Iowa led all others in active generosity.

Under the supervision of Mr. B. F. Tillinghast,

of Davenport, aided by the able pen of Miss Alice French, that State alone raised, and sent in trains across the country from Iowa to New York, one hundred and seventeen thousand bushels of corn and one hundred thousand pounds of flour, which . was loaded onto the " Tynehead," a staunch British ship, and consigned to the port of Riga.

That year we had been notified of an International Conference to be held in Rome. The cus- . tomary appropriation was made by Congress, and again I was appointed delegate. Too much occupied by the relief at home, Dr. Hubbell, also a delegate, went in my place to Rome, and from there reached Riga in time to receive and direct the distribution of the immense cargo of grain throughout Russia.

When Dr. Hubbell reached Riga he learned that two hundred and forty peasants had been waiting on the dock two days, watching and waiting for the ship from America. Not waiting for food, for Riga was not in a famine province, but waiting that they might not miss the opportunity and the honor of unloading the American ship that had brought food to their unfortunate brothers in the

interior. As soon as they could get into the hold
of the ship, one hundred and forty of them began
the unloading. They worked night and day, without rest, determined to unload the entire cargo
themselves, without help. But on the third night
our Consul, Mr. Bornholdt, insisted on their having
a relief of twelve hours, and when the twelve hours
were up they were all in their places again, and remained until the cargo was out, declining to take
any pay for their labor. Twelve women worked
along with them in the same spirit, in the ship and
on the dock, with needles, sewing up the rents in
the bags, to prevent waste in handling, and cooking
meals for the men.

The Mayor of St. Petersburg, in an address on
behalf of that city to American donors, declared:

" The Russian people know how to be grateful.
If up to this day these two great countries, Russia
and the United States, have not only never quar-
reled, but on the contrary wished each other prosperity and strength always, these feelings of sympathy can grow only stronger in the future, both
countries being conscious that in the season of trial
for either it will find in the other cordial succor and

support. And can true friendship be tested if not in the hour of misfortune? "

A peasant of Samara sent to a Russian editor, together with three colored eggs, a letter which he asked to have forwarded to America. The following is an extract from the letter:

" Christ is risen! To the merciful benefactors, the protectors of the poor, the feeders of the starving, the guardians of the orphans—Christ is risen.

" North Americans! May the Lord grant you a peaceful and long life and prosperity to your land, and may your fields be filled with abundant harvest—Christ is risen. Your mercifulness gives us a helping hand. Through your charity you have satisfied the starving. And for your magnificent alms accept from me this humble gift, which I send to the entire American people for your great beneficence, from all the hearts of the poor filled with feelings of joy."

In the gratitude manifested by the Russian Government and people we were glad to feel that a slight return had been made to Russia for past favors in our own peril, and a friendship never broken.

The Department of State at Washington, under date of January 11, 1894, forwarded the following:

"I have to inform you that on November 7, 1893, the American Minister at St. Petersburg received from the nobility of that city, through their Marshal, Count Alexis Bobrinskoy, an address to the people of the United States. This address, which is in the English language, embodies in terms fitly chosen the thanks of the Russian people to the American for the aid sent to their country from our own during the famine period of the past two years. It is beautifully engrossed and its illumination embraces water-color drawings which render it a most attractive work of art.

"The document, which is superbly bound and enclosed in a fine case, was duly forwarded to this city by the American Minister at St. Petersburg, and will be given a conspicuous place in the library of this department."

In so general an uprising of relief no great sum in contributions could be expected from any one source. The Red Cross felt that, if no more, it was glad to be able to pay, by the generous help of the city of Washington, the charter of a ship that conveyed its corn—$12,500—besides several thousands distributed in Russia through Tolstoi and American agents there.

We paid the cost of loading, superintended by Mr. Tillinghast in person, whose financial record shows the exact cost of transportation. All this was done in connection with the State of Iowa. Our home record showed, when all was finished, a field closed with a small balance in our favor, which we had no active call for. By the advice of one of the best personal advisers, bankers, and friends that the Red Cross has ever had, this small sum was placed in bank, in readiness for the next call.

VI

THE SEA ISLAND RELIEF

This little timely provision, advisedly made, was none too much or none too soon.

On the 28th of August, 1893, a hurricane and tidal wave from the direction of the West Indies swept the coast of South Carolina, covering its entire range of Port Royal Islands, sixteen feet below the sea. These islands had thirty-five thousand inhabitants, mainly negroes. At first, it was thought that all must have perished. Later, it was found that only some four or five thousand had been drowned, and that thirty thousand remained with no earthly possession of home, clothing, or food. The few boats not swept away took them over to the mainland in thousands, and calls went out for help. In this emergency Governor Tillman called for the services of the Red Cross, and my note-book has this passage:

" The next night, in a dark, cheerless September mist, I closed my door behind me for ten months, and with three assistants went to the station to meet Senator Butler."

At Columbia we were joined by Governor Tillman, and thus reinforced proceeded to Beaufort. After due examination the work which had been officially placed with us by the Governor was accepted October 1st, and carried on until the following July.

The submerged lands were drained, three hundred miles of ditches made, a million feet of lumber purchased and houses built, fields and gardens planted with the best seed in the United States, and the work all done by the people themselves. The thousands of boxes of clothing received were distributed among them, and we left them in July, 1894, supplies of vegetables for the city of Beaufort.

Free transportation for supplies continued till about March. No provisions in kind were sent from any source after the first four weeks of public excitement. After this all foodstuffs were purchased in Charleston and distributed as rations. Men were compelled to work on the building of their own homes in order to receive rations.

We found them an industrious, grateful class of people, far above the ordinary grade usually met. They largely owned their little homes, and appreciated instruction in the way of improving them. The tender memory of the childlike confidence and obedience of this ebony-faced population is something that time cannot efface from either us or them.

On the third day after our arrival at Beaufort four middle-aged colored men came to the door of the room we had appropriated as an office, and respectfully asked to see "Miss Clare." They were admitted, and I waited to learn what request they would probably make of me. At length the tallest and evidently the leader, said:

"Miss Clare, we knows you doesn't remember us. But we never fo'gits you. We has all of us got somethin' to show you."

Slipping up a soiled, ragged shirtsleeve, he showed me an ugly scar above the elbow, reaching to the shoulder. "Wagner?" I asked.

"Yes, Miss Clare, and you drissed it for me that night, when I crawled down the beach—'cause my leg was broke too," he replied. "And we was all

79

of us there, and you took care of us all and drissed our wounz. I was with Colonel Shaw, and crawled out of the fote. The oth's nevah got in. But we all got to you, Miss Clare. And now you's got to us. We's talked about you a heap o' times, but we nevah 'spected to see you. We's nevah fo'git it, Miss Clare."

One by one they showed their scars. There was very little clothing to hide them—bullet wound and sabre stroke. The memory, dark and sad, stood out before us all. It was a moment not to be forgotten.

Our purchases consisted of meat, mainly dry sides of pork, and grits, or hominy, for eating. For planting, beside the seed contributed and the nine hundred bushels of Irish potatoes, were eighteen hundred bushels of Northern Flint seed corn.

The contributions of food and clothing had been sent to Beaufort, and were in the warehouses of the perplexed committee of its leading citizens. This had naturally drawn all the inhabitants of the scores of desolated islands for fifty miles to Beaufort, until, it is safe to say, that fifteen to twenty thousand refugees had gathered there, living in its streets and waiting to be fed from day to day.

As the food was there they could not be induced to return to the islands. Indeed, there was more often nothing on the islands to return to. The description given by the heads of families and owners, for they had largely owned their homes, gotten on the old-time plantations " 'fo de wah," was this: If all had been swept out to sea and nothing remained, it was described as, " done gone." But if thrown down and parts of the wreck still remained, it was described as " ractified."

A few of the churches, being larger and more strongly built, still remained standing. During the first ten days of our stay it would have been impossible to drive through the principal streets of Beaufort. They were a solid moving mass, crowding as near to the storehouses as possible to get, in spite of the policeman, who kindly held them back.

We sat daily in counsel with the local committee, until seeing that only systematic measures and a decided change could relieve the conditions and

81

render the city safe. We then, on the first of October, decided to accede to the request of the Governor made at first, and take sole charge of the relief.

Our first order was to close every storehouse, both of food and clothing, and inform the people that all distributions would hereafter be made from the islands. It is impossible to convey to the mind of the reader the difficulty of getting into a few intelligent sentences the idea of the means adopted to produce these changes and inaugurate a system that was to restore to active habits of life a body of utterly homeless, demoralized, and ignorant people, equal in numbers to a small new State.

If these little covers would admit the scores of pages of admirably written reports of the officers and helpers on that field, every line replete with interest, that lie here at my hand, it would be an easy and a welcome task to reproduce them entire, and no more than deserved for their faithful and gratuitous labor.

Dr. Egan's report has this passage:

"October 2d came my marching orders. Take charge of the warehouse and stores, make an inventory of them, disperse these men, and rid the city of the demoralizing influence of idle people. The doors are closed and the inventory begun."

The local committee had kindly pointed out the most suitable man to take charge of each community, and to him would be consigned the rations to be distributed to each family and person within his charge, for which receipt and distribution he became as responsible as a merchant.

The goods and rations were at once shipped across the bay to them, or taken on their own boats, if so fortunate as to have one left from the storm. It is needless to say that the multitude followed the food.

In three days there were not people enough left in Beaufort, besides its own, to be hired for a " job of work." Then followed the necessity for material to rebuild the " done gone," and to repair the " ractified " homes.

A million feet of pine lumber was purchased of a leading lumber dealer, shipped down the Combahee River, and delivered at the landings on the islands most convenient of access to the points needed. Each man received his lumber by order and receipt, and was under obligation to build his own house. The work was all performed by themselves. A garden was insisted upon. At first this proposition was resisted as impracticable.

"No use, Mistah—no use—'cause de pig eat it all up."

It was suggested that a fence might be made enclosing at least a quarter of an acre about the house to keep "de pig" out, as we should later send, for planting, the best seed to be obtained in the country.

To this moment our thanks go out to the Agricultural Department at Washington, and the great seed houses of all the North, for the generous donations that served to bring once more into self-sustaining relations this destitute and well-disposed people.

The fact that the building of the fence, and its subsequent keeping in strict repair, had some bearing on the weekly issuance of rations, was evidently not without its influence. There were no poor fences and "de pig" did no damage. But there were such gardens, and of such varieties, as those islands had never before seen.

The earliest crop to strive for, beside the gardens, was the Irish potato, which they had never raised. Nine hundred bushels were purchased from Savannah for planting in February. The difficulty of distributing the potatoes lay in the fact that they would be more likely to find their way into the dinner pot than into the ground. To avoid this the court-yard inside our headquarters was appropriated for the purpose of preparing the potatoes for planting.

Some forty women were hired to come over from the islands and cut potatoes for seed—every " eye " of the potato making a sprout—these distributed to them by the peck, like other seed.

I recall a fine, bright morning in May, when I was told that a woman who had come over from St. Helena in the night, waited at the door to see me. I went to the door to find a tall, bright-looking woman in a clean dress, with a basket on her head, which, after salutation, she lowered and held out to me. There was something over a peck of Early Rose potatoes in the basket—in size from a pigeon's to a pullet's egg. The grateful woman could wait no longer for the potatoes to grow larger, but had dug these, and had come ten miles over the sea, in the night, to bring them to me as a first offering of food of her own raising.

If the tears fell on the little gift as I looked and remembered, no one will wonder or criticise. The potatoes were cooked for breakfast, and " Susie Jane " was invited to partake.

The shores of the mainland had not been exempt from the ravages of the storm and in many instances had suffered like the islands. Some thirty miles above Beaufort was a kind of plantation, with a community of sixty or seventy families of colored people. The property was owned by two elderly white ladies who had not returned since driven away by the storm.

This village was reported to us as in need and demoralized, with no head, scant of food, and its " ractified " houses scarcely affording a shelter.

A representative mulatto man came to tell us. An inspection was made and resulted in this man being put in charge to build up the community. Lumber and food were provided and the people set to work under his charge. From time to time word came to us, and after some months the tall representative came again. He had been asked by the people to come and bring their thanks to the Red Cross for "de home, de gard'n, de pig, and de chick'n dey all has now."

The thanks they had emphasized and proved by the heavy basket that Jackson had carefully brought all the forty miles. It contained seventy-one fresh eggs—the gift of seventy-one families—being a contribution of one egg from each family, from the day or two previous to his leaving on his mission.

Domestic gardens were a new feature among these islanders, whose whole attention had been always given to the raising of the renowned "Sea Island Cotton," the pride of the market, and a just distinction to themselves and the worthy planter. The result of this innovation was that, when we left in July, it was nearly as difficult for a pedestrian to make his way on the narrow sidewalks of Beaufort because of piled-up vegetables for sale from the islands, as it had been in October to pass through the streets because of hungry, idle men and women.

Nothing better illustrates the native good heart

of these people than their kindly interest in and
for each other. Often the young men, without
families, would club together and put up a house
for some lone old " auntie," who had neither family
nor home, and occasionally there seemed to develop
among them an active philanthropist. Of this
type was Jack Owens, who rebuilt his own " done
gone " premises. One day as the field agent was
driving out on some inspection he met Jack walking into town.

His decrepit neighbor's house had burned a few
weeks before, and Jack had gotten lumber and rebuilt the house himself. In describing the utter
devastation, Jack explained that " all de house and
de well was burned "—and he had built another
house and was coming in on foot " for funituh to
funish it." Jack had lost his ox, " a big ox," he
said, in the storm, and now he " hadn't any nuther "
to plow his ground. He pleaded for another—if
it was only " a lil' critter it would grow big "—and
it would help him so much.

The appeal was not to be resisted. Dr. Hubbell
treasures to this day the satisfaction he felt in
procuring something better than the " lil' critter "

88

as reward and encouragement for Jack's active philanthropy.

If any practical woman reading this should try to comprehend what it would be to undertake to clothe and keep clothed thirty thousand human beings for a year, and to do this from the charitable gifts of the people, which gifts had all done more or less service before—often pretty thoroughly "ractified"—this woman will not wonder that sewing societies suggested themselves to us at headquarters.

The women were called together and this suggestion made to them, with the result that an old time "sewing circle" was instituted in every community. Its membership, officers, dues, and regulations were properly established—one-half day in each week devoted by each member to the work in its sewing-rooms, with a woman in charge to prepare it. The clothing was given out to them as received by us. Many a basket came proudly back to show us the difference between " den an' now "— good, strong, firmly mended garments. Ragged coats and pants disappeared from among the men, as no longer " 'spectable fo' de fambly."

Provision was also made that the little girls from
ten years old should attend and be taught to sew.
Many a little dress was selected at headquarters
for them to make over or repair.

I wish I could do fitting justice to the band of
women volunteers who stood by me through those
long months. Some had commenced with me when
society belles, years before, now mistresses of their
own palatial homes; some had come from under the
old historic elms of Boston, and some from the hard-
fought fields of Britain's Africa, and wearing the
Victoria Cross. To them, white and black were
the same, and no toil too hard or too menial.

The money contributed and received for the
entire relief of ten months was thirty thousand five
hundred, and a few additional dollars and cents
which I do not at this moment recall. It aggre-
gated one dollar apiece for the entire maintenance
of thirty thousand persons for ten months.

It is the general custom in this part of the country for the merchants to furnish supplies to their
patrons, and wait until the gathering of the crops
for their pay. But when we left these people at
the beginning of their harvest, not one family in

twenty-five had contracted a debt for supplies: an experience before unknown in their history.

A report was made and passed into the hands of our legal counsellor, who, on seeing that no change could be truthfully made in it, advised that it be not published, as no one would believe it possible to be done, and we would get only distrust and discredit. Having now come to a pass where distrust and discredit are no longer to be feared by the Red Cross, we ourselves are free to make the statement. But back of the hard facts there is compensation.

A half dozen years later, when our negro protégés of the Sea Islands heard of the disaster that had fallen upon Galveston, they at once gathered for aid and sent in their contributions.

" 'Cause dey suffers like we did, and de Red Cross is dar," they said.

Of course I would not permit one dollar of this holy gift to Galveston to go to other than the hands, hard, bony, and black—such as had raised it in their penury. I also wanted it to do more. Searching for the most reliable colored people in the city I found in the superintendent of the colored schools a man who had occupied that place

91

for many years, and who had the respect and confidence of the people of Galveston. I asked him to consult his foremost women teachers, and if it pleased them, to form a society and fit themselves to receive a little money.

In about a week he appeared with his deputation. I informed them that I had a little money from their own people of the Sea Islands for them; that they had been chosen to receive it, because as teachers of the children they would have access to the needs and conditions of the families. I told them that I had desired to do more than merely make a gift for distribution. I wished to plant a tree. I could have given them their peach, which they would eat, enjoy, and throw the pit away. But I wished them to plant the pit, and let it raise other fruit for them, and for that reason I had asked the formation of this society.

They all sat quiet a few moments, the tears were on their faces. At length their president, the school superintendent, spoke for them:

" Miss Barton," he said, " we all appreciate this, and in the name of all I promise you that the pit shall be reverently planted. and I trust the time

92

will come when I can tell you that our tree is not only bearing fruit for ourselves, but for all suffering brethren, as theirs have done for us."

I then handed them the check for $397. The moment seemed sacred when these poor dark figures, struggling toward the light, walked out of my presence. The pit has been successfully planted in Galveston, and we are from time to time informed of its bearing.

VII

LEAVING the Port Royal field past midsummer of 1894, after an absence of nearly a year—at a day's notice—the remainder of the autumn and winter was scarcely less occupied in the details which had been unavoidably overlooked. Before spring our correspondence commenced to enlarge with rumors of Armenian massacres, and so excited and rapid was the increase that, so far as actual labor, consultation, and thought were concerned, we might as well have been on a field of relief.

Unfortunately, the suspicions of the Turkish Government had fallen upon the resident missionaries, both English and American, as favoring the views and efforts of its anarchistic population, or the " young Turks," as they were designated. This had the effect of placing the missionaries in danger, confining them strictly to their own quar-

94

ters, preventing all communication and the receiving of any funds sent them from abroad.

England had a large waiting fund which it could not distribute, and appealed to the American Missionary Boards of Boston and New York, to find them equally powerless. The need of funds among the missionaries throughout Turkey was getting painfully urgent, and as a last resort it was suggested from Constantinople that the Red Cross be asked to open the way.

A written request from the Rev. Judson Smith, D.D., of Boston, was nearly identical with one received by us from Mr. Spencer Trask, of New York, who with others was about to form a national Armenian relief committee, to be established in that city.

Following these communications, both of these eminent gentlemen, Mr. Smith and Mr. Trask, came in person to urge our compliance with their request that the Red Cross accept the charge and personally undertake the doubtful and dangerous task of distributing the waiting funds among the missionaries in Turkey.

As Mr. Trask was to take the lead in the forma-

tion of a committee for the raising of funds, his
interest was naturally paramount, and his argu-
ments in favor of our acceptance were wellnigh
irresistible. Immediate action on the part of some
one was imperative. Human beings were starving,
and could not be reached. Thousands of towns
and villages had not been heard from since the
massacres, and only the Red Cross could have any
hope of reaching them. No one else was prepared
for field work; it had its force of trained field
workers. Turkey was one of the signatory powers
to the Red Cross Treaty. Thus it was hoped and
believed that she would the more readily accept
its presence.

These are mere examples of the reasons urged
by the ardent advocates of the proposed committee, until at length we came to consider its
acceptance, on conditions which must be clearly
understood. First, we must not be expected to
take any part in, or to be made use of, in the raising of funds—one of our fundamental rules being
never to ask for funds—we did not do it for
ourselves.

Second, there must be perfect unanimity between themselves. We must be assured that every one wanted us to go. Our part would be hard enough then; and finally we must be sure they had some funds to distribute.

Of the amount of these funds no mention was made by us, and I remember a feeling of good-natured amusement as I heard the officers of this untried effort at raising funds speak of " millions." It was easy to discern that they were more accustomed to the figures of a banking establishment than a charity organization dependent on the raising of funds. They were likely to be disappointed. In reality, the amount, so there were something to go with, made very little difference to us, as we were merely to place what was entrusted to us where most needed, and when that was done we had but to return. We never named any amount as preferable to us.

The means resorted to in raising the funds were unfortunate. In the great public meetings called for that purpose the utmost indiscretion prevailed in regard to language applied to Turkey and the Turkish Government. This aroused the indignation of the Turkish officials, who very reasonably

97

took measures to have our entrance into Turkey forbidden.

A date of sailing, however, had been given Mr. Trask, and his committee, feeling that any change would be detrimental to their efforts, no change was made, and we sailed on time, to find in England no permission, and further efforts necessary. With time and patience the troublesome effects of these mistakes were overcome, and Constantinople was reached, and a heavenly welcome by the harassed missionaries awaited us.

The first step was to procure an introduction to the Turkish Government, which had in one sense refused to see me. Accompanied by the American Minister, Hon. A. W. Terrell, and his premier interpreter, Gargiulo, one of the most experienced diplomatic officers in Constantinople, I called by appointment upon Tewfik Pasha, the Turkish Minister of Foreign Affairs, or Minister of State. To those conversant with the personages connected with Turkish affairs, I need not say that Tewfik Pasha is probably the foremost man of the government—a manly man, with a kind, fine face, and genial, polished manners. Educated abroad, with

98

advanced views on general subjects, he impresses one as a man who would sanction no wrong it was in his power to avert.

Mr. Terrell's introduction was most appropriate and well expressed, bearing with strong emphasis upon the suffering condition of the people of the interior, in consequence of the massacres, the great sympathy of the people of America, and giving assurance that our objects were purely humanitarian, having neither political, racial, nor religious significance.

The Pasha listened most attentively to Mr. Terrell, thanked him, and said that this was well understood, that they knew the Red Cross and its president. Turning to me he repeated: " We know you, Miss Barton; have long known you and your work. We would like to hear your plans for relief and what you desire."

I proceeded to state our plans for relief, which, if not carried out at this time, the suffering in Armenia, unless we had been misinformed, would shock the entire civilized world. None of us knew from personal observation, as yet, the full need of assistance, but had reason to believe it very great.

99

If my agents were permitted to go, such need as they found they would be prompt to relieve. On the other hand, if they did not find the need existing there, none would leave the field so gladly as they. There would be no respecting of persons— humanity alone would be their guide. "We have," I added, "brought only ourselves; no correspondent has accompanied us, and we shall have none, and shall not go home to write a book on Turkey. We are not here for that. Nothing shall be done in any concealed manner. All dispatches which we send will go openly through your own telegraph, and I should be glad if all that we shall write could be seen by your government. I can not, of course, say what its character will be, but can vouch for its truth, fairness, and integrity, and for the conduct of every leading man who shall be sent. I shall never counsel or permit a sly or underhand action with your government, and you will pardon me, Pasha, if I say I shall expect the same treatment in return—such as I give I shall expect to receive."

Almost without a breath he replied: "And you shall have it. We honor your position and your wishes shall be respected. Such aid and protection as we are able, we shall render." .

I then asked if it were necessary for me to see other officials. " No," he replied, " I speak for my government," and with cordial good wishes our interview closed.

I never spoke personally with this gentleman again, all further business being officially transacted through the officers of our legation. Yet I can truly say, as I have said of my first meeting with our matchless band of missionary workers, that here commenced an acquaintance which proved invaluable, and here were given pledges of mutual faith, of which not a word was ever broken on either side.

The Turkish Government, when once it came to understand American methods and enthusiasm, was forgiving and kind to us. No obstruction was ever placed in our way. Our five expeditions passed through Armenian Turkey from sea to sea, distributing whatever was needed, repairing the destroyed machines, enabling the people to make tools to harvest their grain, thus averting a famine; providing medical help and food as well for

thousands of sick; setting free the frightened inhabitants, and returning them to the villages from
which they had fled for their lives; restoring all
missionary freedom that had been interrupted;
establishing a more kindly feeling toward them on
the part of the government; and through all this,
we had never one unpleasant transaction with any
person of whatever name or race.

While our expeditions were getting ready to go
out by the Black Sea, a request was brought to
me by Dr. Washburn, of Robert College, from Sir
Philip Currie, the British Ambassador at Constantinople, asking if I could not be "persuaded"
to turn my expedition through the Mediterranean,
rather than the Black Sea, in order to reach Mirash
and Zeitoun, where the foreign consuls were at the
moment convened. They had gotten word to him
that ten thousand people in those two cities were
down with four distinct epidemics—typhoid and
typhus fevers, dysentery and smallpox—that the
victims were dying in overwhelming numbers, and
that there was not a physician among them, all being either sick or dead, with no medicine and little
food.

This was not a case for " persuasion," but of heartfelt thanks from us all, that Sir Philip had remembered to call us, whom he had never met. But here was a hindrance. The only means of conveyance from Constantinople to Alexandretta were coasting boats, belonging to different nationalities, which left only once in two weeks, and irregularly at that. Transport for our goods was secured on the first boat to leave, the goods taken to the wharf at Galata, and at the latest moment, in order to give time, a request was made to the government for *teskeres*, or traveling permits, for Dr. J. B. Hubbell and assistants. To our surprise they were granted instantly, but by some delay on the part of the messenger sent for them they reached a moment too late. The boat left a little more promptly, taking with it our relief goods, and leaving the men on the dock to receive their permits only when the boat was beyond recall. It was really the fault of no one.

With the least possible delay Dr. Hubbell secured passage by the first boat at Smyrna, and a fortunate chance boat from there took him to Alexandretta, via Beyrout and Tripoli, Syria.

The goods arrived in safety, and two other of our assistants, whom we had called by cable from America—Edward M. Wistar and Charles King Wood—were also passed over to the same point with more goods. There, caravans were fitted out to leave over the—to them—unknown track to Aintab, as a first base. From this point the reports of these three gentlemen made to me will be living witnesses. They tell their own modest tales of exposure, severe travel, hard work, and hardship, of which no word of complaint has ever passed their lips. There have been only gratitude and joy, that they could do something in a cause at once so great and so terrible.

While this was in progress, a dispatch came to me at Constantinople from Dr. Shepard of Aintab, whose tireless hands had done the work of a score of men, saying that fevers, both typhoid and typhus, of the most virulent nature, had broken out in Arabkir, two or three days north of Harpoot; could I send doctors and help? Passing the word on to Dr. Hubbell at Harpoot, prompt and courageous action was taken by him. It is something to say that from a rising pestilence with a score of deaths daily, in five weeks, himself and his assistants left the city in a normally healthful condition, the mortality ceasing at once under their care and treatment.

During this time the medical relief for the cities of Zeitoun and Marash was in charge of Dr. Ira Harris, of Tripoli, who reached there March 18th. The report of the consuls had placed the number of deaths from the four contagious diseases at one hundred a day. This would be quite probable when it is considered that ten thousand were smitten with the prevailing diseases, and that added to this were the crowded condition of the patients, the thousands of homeless refugees who had flocked from their forsaken villages, the lack of all comforts, of air, cleanliness, and a state of prolonged starvation.

Dr. Harris's first report to me was that he was obliged to set the soup kettles boiling and feed his patients before medicine could be retained. My reply was a draft for two hundred liras (something over eight hundred dollars) with the added dispatch: " Keep the pot boiling; let us know your wants." The further reports show from this time

8   105

an astonishingly small number of deaths. The utmost care was taken by all our expeditions to prevent the spread of the contagion and there is no record of its ever having been carried out of the cities, where it was found, either at Zeitoun, Marash, or Arabkir. Lacking this precaution, it might well have spread throughout all Asia Minor, as was greatly feared by the anxious people.

On the twenty-fourth of May, Dr. Harris reported the disease as overcome. His stay being no longer needed, he returned to his great charge in Tripoli, with the record of a medical work and success behind him never surpassed if ever equaled. The lives he had saved were enough to gain Heaven's choicest diadem. Never has America cause to be more justly proud and grateful than when its sons and daughters in foreign lands perform deeds of worth like that.

The closing of the medical fields threw our entire force into the general relief of the vilayet of Harpoot, which the relieving missionaries had well named their " bottomless pit."

The apathy to which the state of utter nothingness, together with their grief and fear, had reduced the inhabitants, was by no means the smallest difficulty to be overcome. Here was realized the great danger felt by all—that of continued alms-giving, lest they settle down into a condition of pauperism, and thus finally starve, from the inability of the world at large to feed them. The presence of a strange body of friendly working people, coming thousands of miles to help them, awakened a hope and stimulated the desire to help themselves.

It was a new experience that these strangers *dared* to come to them. Although the aforetime home lay a heap of stone and sand, and nothing belonging to it remained, still the land was there, and when seed to plant the ground and the farming utensils and cattle were brought to work it with, the faint spirit revived, the weak, hopeless hands unclasped, and the farmer stood on his feet again.

When the cities could no longer provide the spades, hoes, plows, picks and shovels, and the crude iron and steel to make these was purchased and taken to them, the blacksmith found again his fire and forge and traveled weary miles with his bellows on his back. The carpenter again swung his hammer and drew his saw. The broken and scattered spinning-wheels and looms from under the storms and *débris* of winter again took form and motion, and the fresh bundles of wool, cotton, flax, and hemp in the waiting widow's hand brought hopeful visions of the revival of industries which should not only clothe but feed.

At length, in early June, the great grain-fields of Diarbekir, Farkin, and Harpoot valleys, planted the year before, grew golden and bowed their heavy spear-crowned heads in waiting for the sickle. But no sickles were there, no scythes, not even knives. It was a new and sorry sight for our full-handed American farming men to see those poor, hard Asiatic hands trying, by main strength, to break the tough straw or pull it by the roots. This state of things could not continue, and their sorrow and pity gave place to joy when they were able to drain the cities of Harpoot and Diarbekir of harvest tools, and turned the work of all the village blacksmiths on to the manufacture of sickles and scythes, and of flint workers upon the rude threshing machines.

They have told me since their return that the

pleasantest memories left to them were of those great valleys of golden grain, bending and falling before the harvesters, men and women, each with the new, sharp sickle or scythe, the crude threshing planks, the cattle trampling out the grain, and the gleaners in the rear as in the days of Abraham and Moab. God grant that somewhere among them was a kind-hearted king of the harvest who gave orders to let some sheaves fall.

Even while this saving process was going on another condition no less imperative arose. These fields must be replanted or starvation must be simply delayed. Only the strength of their old-time teams of oxen could break up the hard sod and prepare for the fall sowing. Not an animal—ox, cow, horse, goat, or sheep—had been left. All had been driven to the Kourdish Mountains. When Mr. Wood's telegram came, calling for a thousand oxen for the hundreds of villages, I thought of our not rapidly swelling bank account, and all that was needed everywhere else, and replied accordingly.

When in return came the telegram from the Rev. Dr. Gates, president of Harpoot College, the live, active, practical man of affairs, whose judgment no one could question, saying that the need of oxen was imperative, that unless the ground could be plowed before it dried and hardened it could not be done at all, and the next harvest would be lost, also that " Mr. Wood's estimate was moderate," the financial secretary was directed to send a draft for five thousand liras (twenty-two thousand dollars) to the care of the Rev. Dr. Gates, to be divided among the three expeditions for the purchase of cattle and the progress of the harvest of 1897.

As the sum sent would be immediately applied, the active services of the men would be no longer required, and directions went with the remittance to report in person at Constantinople.

Unheard-of toil, care, hard riding day and night, with risk of life, were all involved in the carrying out of that order. Among the uncivilized and robber bands of Kourds, the cattle that had been stolen and driven off must be picked up, purchased, and brought back to the waiting farmer's field. There were routes so dangerous that a brigand chief was selected by those understanding the situation as the safest escort for our men. Perhaps the greatest danger encountered was in the region of Farkin, beyond Diarbekir, where the official escort had not been waited for, and the leveled musket of the faithless guide told the difference.

At length the task was accomplished. One by one the expeditions closed and withdrew, returning by Sivas and Samsoun, and coming out by the Black Sea. With the return of the expeditions we closed the field. But contributors would be glad to know that subsequent to this, before leaving Constantinople, funds from both the New York and Boston committees came to us amounting to about fifteen thousand dollars. This was happily placed with Mr. W. W. Peet, treasurer of the Board of Foreign Missions at Stamboul, to be used subject to our order; and with our concurrence it was employed in the building of little houses in the interior, as a winter shelter and protection, where all had been destroyed.

The appearance of our men on their arrival at Constantinople confirmed the impression that they had not been recalled too soon. They had gone

111

out through the snows and ice of winter, and without change or rest had come back through the scorching suns of midsummer—five months of rough, uncivilized life, faring and sharing with their beasts of burden, well-nigh out of communication with the civilized world, but never out of danger. It seemed but just to themselves and to others who might need them, that change and rest be given them.

It would scarcely be permissible to express in words the obligation to our American Minister, Hon. A. W. Terrell, at Constantinople, without whose unremitting care and generous aid our work could not have been accomplished. And, indeed, so many were the duties of that difficult and delicate field that it seemed the help of no one hand or heart could be spared. We felt that we had them all; from the palace of the Sultan to beloved Robert College, from the American Legation to the busy rooms of the American Board, with its masterly treasurer, Peet, were the same outstretched hands of protection and care for our little band.

They knew we had taken our lives in our hands

112

to come to them, and with no thought of ourselves. We had done the best we knew to accomplish the mission so persistently sought of us in our own country.

That our work had been acceptable to those who received its results, we knew. They had never failed to *make* us know. If also acceptable to Him who gave us the courage, protection, and strength to perform it, we need care for little more.

Funds to the total amount of $116,326.01 were cabled us by Mr. Spencer Trask's committee, all of which were placed in the hands of Mr. W. W. Peet, treasurer of the missionary board at Constantinople. All proper receipts were given and taken, and feeling that we had faithfully and successfully accomplished the work we had been asked to perform, we closed the field, and prepared to return to America.

Some days of physical rest were needful for the men of the expeditions after reaching Constantinople before commencing their journey of thousands of miles for home, worn as they were by exposure and incessant labor—physical and mental. I need not attempt to say with what gratitude I

113

welcomed back these weary, brown-faced men and officers from a field so difficult and so perilous; none the less did the gratitude go out to my faithful and capable secretary, who had toiled early and late, never leaving for a day, striving with tender heart that all should go well.

And when the first greetings were over, the full chorus of manly voices—" Home Again," " Sweet Land of Liberty," " Nearer My God to Thee "—that rolled out through the open windows of the Red Cross headquarters in Constantinople fell on the listening ears of Christian and Moslem alike, and though the tones were new and strange, all felt that to some one, somewhere, they meant more than the mere notes of music.

VIII

CUBA

1898

On our return to " civilization " we were re-
joiced to find that as a result of our three months'
labors, the former tumult of Armenia had died
away into a peaceful echo, but a new murmur fast
growing to clamor had taken its place. Cuba had entered the ceaseless arena of American, gladiatorial,
humanitarian contest. The cruelties of the recon-
centrado system of warfare had become apparent,
and methods of relief were uppermost in the minds
of all persons.

These methods were twofold and might well be
classed under two distinct heads: those who for
mere pity's sake sought simple relief; those who
with a further forecast sought the removal of a
cause as well as its effect, and " Cuba Libre " was
its muffled cry. They asked money for arms as
well as bread, and the struggle between the two

115

held the country in a state of perplexed contradiction for months running into years.

Our great-hearted President asked simple aid and was distressed at the doubtful response. At length he suggested and we proffered the aid of the Red Cross on a call to the country, and the establishment of the " Central Cuban Relief Committee " in New York, within three days, was the result.

The activity and success of that committee are too fresh in the minds of all our people to require the smallest description from me. Too much praise can not be given to our Auxiliary Societies from the Atlantic to the Pacific for the splendid work in the camps at home, in Cuba, Porto Rico, and in the care of our soldiers in transit to the Philippines. Their full and complete reports show the great work accomplished. The memory of the work of the busy men and tireless women who joined heart and hand in this Heaven-sent task still brings tears to the eyes of a nation at its recall.

The service assigned me by our anxious President, and gladly accepted, was the distribution

116

on the pitiful fields of Cuba. These scenes I would not recall. The starving mothers and motherless babes, the homelessness and squalor, the hopelessness and despair, are beyond all words and all conception, save to those who saw and lived among them. It is past and let it rest.

Then followed the declaration of hostilities, the blockade, the fleets of war, and the stately, glistening white ships of relief that dotted the sea—our navy after forty years of peace again doing service in its own waters—and among them one inconspicuous, black-hulled sea-going craft, laden with food for the still famishing reconcentrados, when they could be reached.

Day after day, in its weary, waiting cruise, it watched out for an opening to that closed-in suffering island, till at length the thunder of the guns, Siboney, San Juan, opened the track, and the wounded troops of our own army, hungering on their own fields, were the reconcentrados of the hour.

Tampa became the gathering-point of the army. Its camps filled like magic, first with regulars, then volunteers, as if the fiery torch of Duncraigen had

117

spread over the hills and prairies of America. The great ships gathered in the waters, the transports, with decks dark with human life, passed in and out, and the battleships of the sea held ever their commanding sway. It seemed a strange thing, this gathering for war. Thirty years of peace had made it strange to all save the veterans of the days of the old war, long passed into history. Could it be possible that we were to learn this anew? Were men again to fall, and women weep? Were the youth of this generation to gain that experience their fathers had gained, to live the war-lives they had lived, and die the deaths they had died?

At length the fleet moved on, and we prepared to move with, or rather after it. The quest on which it had gone, and the route it had taken, bordered something on the mystery shrouding the days when Sherman marched to the sea. Where were the Spanish ships? What would be the result when found and met? Where were we to break that Cuban wall and let us in?

Always present in our minds were the food we carried, the willing hands that waited, and the perishing thousands that needed. We knew the great hospital ships were fitting for the care of the men of both Army and Navy. Surely they could have no need of us.

We had taken possession of our ship at Key West on the 29th of April. It was now the 20th of June and the national records of two countries at least will always give the history of those days. It is our part to keep as clearly, truthfully, and kindly as possible, the record of the little that fell to us to perform in this great drama.

Weighing anchor at Key West the State of Texas steamed for the open Caribbean, we having first taken the official advice of Commodore Remy to find Admiral Sampson and report to him.

Sunrise of the twenty-fifth gave us our first view of the water at Santiago. Our transports and battle-ships were gathered there. The advice of Admiral Sampson was that we proceed to Guantanamo, where the marines had made a landing and were camped on the shore. There had been some fighting at Guantanamo. The naval hospital ship Solace was there.

Whoever has enjoyed this quiet, sheltered harbor, protected on three sides by beautiful wooded hills, will not require to be reminded of it. At six o'clock our anchor sunk in the deep, still waters and we had time to look about and see the beginning of the war. The marines were camped along the brow of a hill. On our right a camp of Cubans, and all about us the great war-ships with their guns, which told of forthcoming trouble. Captain McCalla, who was in command of Guantanamo, had sent his compliments and a launch, leading us in to our place of anchorage. The courtesies of the navy so early commenced at Key West were continued throughout the war.

By invitation of Commander Dunlap our entire company visited the Solace the following day. If that beautiful ship or its management had left room on the records of our country's meed of gratitude, for more words of appreciative praise, I should be glad to speak them. Only those familiar with the earliest history of the Red Cross in our country, and the methods by which our navy alone—of all the Red Cross nations—had gained even an approximately legal place, can judge what the sight of that first naval relief ship in American waters was to me. It brought back

120

so vividly the memory of the day in 1881 when President Arthur called me to him to carefully explain the conditions of the treaty which he had just signed, and that, Congress having generously included the navy in its treaty for war, he would provide to hold it carefully until the probable widening of the original treaty would include the *navies* of the world, as well as the armies.

Before the day closed news came to us of a serious character. The daring Rough Riders had been hardly dealt by. Hamilton Fish and Allyn Capron had been killed, and the wounded needed help. Wherever they might be, it must be possible to reach them, and it was decided that no time be lost. Our men commenced work in the hold of the ship to get at medical supplies and dressings, and the captain took his orders. I find in my diary at the close of that day the following paragraph: " It is the Rough Riders we go to, and the relief may be also rough, but it will be *ready.* A better body of helpers could scarcely be gotten together."

Nine o'clock of the same night found us at Siboney, which can scarcely be called a harbor, for it has no anchorage. The next morning at daybreak we stood on deck to see the soldiers filing up over the hill, in heavy marching order, forming in lines by ones and twos, winding up, in and out among the hills, higher and higher. As we watched them they were a moving line trailing on toward the clouds, till lost in the mist, and we could only think, as we looked at them, on how many and on which, is set the mark of death? He knew no more than we—poor fellow—and with his swinging, steady gait, toils up and up and waits for—he knows not what.

The hospitals, both American and Cuban, located on the shore just to the right of us, were visited by our men that same evening. Some of their surgeons called on us. All seemed interested in the Red Cross, but none thought that a woman nurse would be in place in a soldiers' hospital—indeed, very much out of place. I suggested that that decision was hard for me, for I had spent a great deal of time in soldiers' hospitals myself. They appeared to understand that perfectly, but there seemed to be a *later* line which could not be crossed.

The Cubans who had just come into camp ex-

122

pressed a desire for any assistance we could give them. They would be glad to have the Red Cross Sisters in their little hospital, but begged us to wait just a day until it could be put in better order. The Sisters were not the persons to grant that day of preparation.

On the contrary they at once went to work, thoroughly cleaned the little three-room building— Garcia's abandoned headquarters, to be used as a hospital—and when the day closed the transformation showed clean rooms, clean cots, and the grateful occupants wondering whether Heaven itself could be more comfortable, or anything more desirable than the palatable food prepared for them by the Sisters.

Three days later the following letter was received:

" To Miss CLARA BARTON, President,
        " American National Red Cross:
    " I have the honor to request your assistance in caring for the patients in a so-called hospital near the landing at this point.
    " The orders are to the effect that all patients now under treatment on the shore shall be trans-

ferred to the Iroquois and Olivette, but the facilities for carrying out this order are apparently inadequate. In order that the division hospital may remain unhampered for the care of the wounded in the engagement about to take place, it is necessary for me to request this favor of you, and I trust that you may find it possible to comply with said request.

"Your obedient servant,
"LOUIS A. LE GARDE,
"Major and Surgeon, U. S. A., Commanding Hospital."

To this the following reply was immediately returned:

"Steamship State of Texas,
"SIBONEY, SANTIAGO DE CUBA, *June* 30, 1898.
"DR. LOUIS A. LE GARDE,
"Major and Surgeon, U. S. A., Commanding Hospital.

"Major: Permit me to express the pleasure given me by your letter inviting the assistance of the persons here under my direction in the care of the sick and wounded of the engagement about to take place. Although not here as a hospital ship by any means—not legitimately fitted for the work

124

—still we have some hospital supplies, a few intelligent workers, skill, experience, the willingness to serve, the readiness to obey, and I believe the true spirit of the Red Cross, that seeks to help humanity wherever its needs exist. I send them to you in the hope that they may be of service.

" Cordially yours,

" CLARA BARTON,

" President, American National Red Cross."

Our surgeons and assistants went on shore, where Dr. Le Garde and Dr. Lesser secured a small house, and in a few hours this had undergone the same transformation and by the same hands as the Cuban hospital. The Red Cross flag was hoisted, Dr. Lesser placed in charge, and scores of our soldiers who had been lying on the filthy floors of an adjacent building, with no food but army rations, were carried over, placed in clean cots, and given proper food. From that on, no distinction was made, the Red Cross flag floating over both the American and Cuban hospitals.

A few feet away, all the available army tents were put up as additional accommodation for the " wounded in the engagement about to take place."

It did take place the following day, and, as will be
well remembered, in those two days, Friday and
Saturday, the first and second of July, the tents
were more than filled with wounded in the battle
of San Juan Hill. Three of the five Sisters went
into the operating tent, and with the surgeons
worked for thirty hours with only a few moments'
rest now and then for a cup of coffee and a cracker
or piece of bread. We heard nothing more about
a woman nurse being out of place in a soldiers'
hospital.

On Saturday evening, the second day of the San
Juan battle, a slip of paper with these penciled
words was brought to the door of the hospital:

" Send food, medicines, anything. Seize wagons
from the front for transportation.

"SHAFTER."

The call for help was at once sent over to the
State of Texas, and we worked all night getting
out supplies and sending them ashore with a force
of Cubans, only too glad to work for food.

I wish I could make apparent how difficult a
thing it was to get supplies from our ship to the

shore in a surf which, after ten o'clock in the morning, allowed no small boats to touch even the bit of a pier that was run out without breaking either the one or the other, and nothing in the form of a lighter save two dilapidated flat-boat pontoons. These had been broken and cast away by the engineer corps, picked up by ourselves, mended by the Cubans, and put in condition to float alongside of our ship, and receive perhaps three or four tons of material. This must then be rowed or floated out to the shore, run onto the sand as far as possible, the men jumping into the water from knee to waist deep, pulling the boat up from the surf, and getting the material on land. And this was what was meant by loading the " seized wagons from the front " and getting food to the wounded. After ten o'clock in the day even this was impossible, and we must wait until the calm of three o'clock next morning to commence work again and go through the same struggle to get something to load the wagons for that day. Our supplies had been gotten ashore, and among the last, rocking and tossing in our little boat, went ourselves, landing on the pier, which by that time was break-

ing in two, escaping a surf which every other moment threatened to envelop one from feet to head,
we reached the land.

Our "seized" wagons had already gone on,
loaded with our best hospital supplies—meal, flour,
condensed milk, malted milk, tea, coffee, sugar,
dried fruits, canned fruits, canned meats, and such
other things as we had been able to get out in the
haste of packing—entirely filling the two wagons
already in advance.

An ambulance had been spoken of. We waited
a little while by the roadside, but the ambulance
did not appear. Then, halting a wagon loaded
with bales of hay, we begged a ride of the driver,
and our little party, Dr. and Mrs. Gardner, James
McDowell, and myself, took our seats on the hay
and made our way to the front, Dr. Hubbell following afoot. Four hours' ride brought us to the
First Division Hospital of the Fifth Army Corps
—General Shafter's headquarters.

The sight that met us on going into the so-called
hospital grounds was something indescribable.
The land was perfectly level; no drainage whatever; covered with long, tangled grass; skirted by

trees, brush, and shrubbery; a few little dog-tents not much larger than could have been made of an ordinary table-cloth thrown over a short rail, and under these lay huddled together the men fresh from the field or from the operating-tables, with no covering over them save such as had clung to them through their troubles, and in the majority of cases no blanket under them.

Those who had come from the tables, having been compelled to leave all the clothing they had, as too wet, muddy, and bloody to be retained, were entirely nude, lying on the stubble grass, the sun fitfully dealing with them, sometimes clouding over and again streaming out in a blaze above them. Fortunately, among our supplies were some bolts of unbleached cotton, and this we cut in sheet lengths, and the men of our party went about and covered the poor fellows, who lay there with no shelter either from the elements or the eyes of the passers-by.

A half dozen bricks laid about a yard apart, a couple of pieces of wagon-tire laid across these, so low and so near the ground that no fire of any strength or benefit could be made—the bits

of wet wood put under crosswise, with the smoke
streaming a foot out on either side, two kettles of
coffee or soup, and a small frying-pan with some
meat in it—appeared to be the cook-house for these
men. They told us there were about eight hundred
men under the tents and lying in the grass, and
more constantly coming in.

After a few moments' consultation as to the best
methods to be pursued, we too gathered stones and
bricks and constructed a longer, higher fireplace,
got more wagon-tires, found the water, and soon
our great agate kettles of seven and ten gallons
were filled.

The rain, that had been drizzling more or less
all day, increased. Our supplies were taken from
the wagons, a piece of tarpaulin found to protect
them, and as the fire began to blaze and the water
to heat, Mrs. Gardner and I found the way into
the bags and boxes of flour, salt, milk, and meal,
and got material for the first gallons of gruel. I
had not thought to ever make gruel again over a
camp-fire. I can not say how far it carried me
back in the lapse of time, or really where, or who
I felt that I was.

It did not seem to be me, and still I seemed to know how to do it.

When the bubbling contents of our kettle thickened and grew white with the condensed milk, and we began to give it out—putting it into the hands of men detailed as nurses, and our own men, to take around to the poor sufferers, shivering and naked in the rain—I felt that perhaps it was not in vain that history had repeated itself. When the nurses came back and told us of the surprise with which it was received, and the tears that rolled down the sun-burned, often bloody face, into the cup as the poor fellow drank his hot gruel, and asked where it came from, who sent it, and said it was the first food he had tasted in three days (for they had gone into the fight hungry), I felt that it was again the same old story and wondered what gain there had been in the last thirty years.

The fires burned, the gruel steamed and boiled— bucket after bucket went out—until those eight hundred men had each a cup of gruel and knew that he could have another and as many as he wanted. The day waned, the darkness came, and still the men were unsheltered, uncovered, naked,

131

and wet—scarcely a groan, no word of complaint
—no man said he was not well treated.

The operating-tables were full of the wounded.
Man after man was taken off, brought on his litter
and laid beside other men, and something given
him to keep the little life in his body that seemed
fast oozing out. All night it went on. It grew
cold—for naked men bitter cold—before morning. We had no blankets, nothing to cover them,
only the strips of cotton cloth.

Early in the morning ambulances started, and
such of the wounded as could be loaded in were
taken to be carried back over that rough, pitiless
road, down to Siboney, to the hospitals there—
that we had done the best we could toward fitting
up—where our hundred cots, hundred and fifty
blankets had gone, cups, spoons, and delicacies,
that would help to strengthen these poor, fainting
men, if they could get there, and where also the
Sisters would care for them.

They brought man after man, stretcher after
stretcher, to the waiting ambulances, and they took
out seventeen who had died in the night, unat-
tended, save by the nurse.

More supplies arrived, and this time came large tarpaulins, more utensils, more food, and more things to make it a little comfortable. We removed our first kitchens across the road, up alongside the headquarter tent of Major Wood, in charge of the camp. Words can not do justice to his kind-hearted generosity. He strove in every way to do all that could be done, and the night before had given us a small tent in which we had huddled from the pouring rain, for a couple of hours, in the middle of the night, the water rushing through like a rivulet.

The tarpaulins were put over supplies, a new fireplace made near us—magnificent in its dimensions—shelter given for boxes and barrels that by this time had accumulated about us, and there was even something that looked like a table, on which Mrs. Gardner prepared her delicacies.

Early in the day there came to our improvised headquarters an officer in khaki uniform showing hard service, and a bandanna handkerchief hanging from his hat, to protect the back of his head and neck from the fierce rays of the sun.

It was Colonel Roosevelt, and we were very glad

to meet the gallant leader of the " Rough Riders."
After a few moments conversation he said:

" I have some sick men with the regiment who
refuse to leave it. They need such delicacies as you
have here, which I am ready to pay for out of my
own pocket. Can I buy them from the Red
Cross? "

" Not for a million dollars," Dr. Gardner replied.

" But my men need these things," he said, his
tone and face expressing anxiety. " I think a
great deal of my men. I am proud of them."

" And we know they are proud of you, Colonel.
But we can't sell Red Cross supplies," answered
Dr. Gardner.

" Then, how can I get them? I must have
proper food for my sick men," he said.

" Just ask for them, Colonel," replied Dr. Gardner.

" Oh," he said, his face suddenly lighting up
with a bright smile; " then I do ask for them."

" All right, Colonel; what is your list? "

The list included malted milk, condensed milk,
oatmeal, cornmeal, canned fruits, dried fruits, rice,

tea, chocolate, and even prepared beefsteak and vegetables, and other things good for men who could not eat army rations.

"Now, Colonel, when will you send for these supplies?" asked Dr. Gardner. "They will be ready any time."

"Lend me a sack and I'll take them right along," he answered with characteristic decision.

Mrs. Gardner at once looked up a sack, and when filled it must have held a good many pounds of supplies. Before we had recovered from our surprise, the incident was closed by the future President of the United States slinging the big sack over his shoulders, striding off, and out of sight through the jungle.

The gruel still remained the staple, but malted milk, chocolate, rice, and tea had come in, and little by little various things were added by which our *menage* quite resembled a hotel. The wounded were still being taken away by ambulance and wagon, assorted and picked over like fruit. Those who would bear transportation were taken away, the others left where they were. By the third day our patients seemed strong enough that we might risk giving them food as solid as rice, and the great kettles were filled with that, cooked soft, mixed with condensed and malted milk. The number of wounded grew less day by day, and better care could be taken of them.

At Siboney, the great needs of the hour were met by the little band of surgeons and nurses, working night and day. The following is from a letter in the Times-Herald, now Record-Herald, of Chicago, by Miss Janet Jennings, who volunteered her service in the hospital. One gets from this simple, direct picture, a better appreciation of that heroism which lives after excitement, which survives the rush and shouting of assault, which is sustained without comradeship:

"SIBONEY, *July* 8, 1898.

"Above hospital tents Red Cross flags are flying, and here is the real life—the suffering and heroism. Everybody who can do even so little as carry a cup of water lends willing hands to help the wounded. Most of the wounded are from the first day's engagement, when the infantry was ordered to lead the attack on Santiago, instead of using the artillery.

136

"And it all came at once—a quick blow—with little or no preparation to meet it. I mentioned in a former letter the lack of preparation on the part of the army to care for the sick. There was then almost nothing—no cots, bedding or proper food, for less than one hundred sick men.

"Two days later, when the wounded came in, the needs of the hour were overwhelming. The situation can not be described. Thousands of our men had been hurried to the front to fight. It was well understood that it would be a hard fight. The dead would need only burial, but the wounded would need care. And yet, with the exception of a limited number of stretchers, a medicine-chest and a few bandages, no preparation had been made —neither cots nor food—practically no hospital supplies.

"It is not strange that surgeons were desperate and nurses distressed. The force of each was wholly inadequate. The exact number of wounded may never be known. But the estimate at this time is about 1,000 wounded—some 1,500 killed and wounded.

"Wounded men who made their way down on foot eight miles over the rough, hilly road will never know just how their strength held out. Others were brought down in army wagons by

10   137

the load, as few ambulances were at hand. Fortunately, there were some tents here that had been used by troops before going to the front. Under these hay was spread and covered with blankets, and the improvised hospital was ready. One tent was taken for operating-tables, and the work of surgeons and nurses began. They worked night and day for forty-eight hours, with only brief intervals for coffee and hard-tack.

"Wounded men had to wait for hours before bullets could be extracted and wounds dressed. But there was no word of complaint—only silent, patient suffering, borne with a courage that was sublime. As the wounded continued to come in, tent-room gave out, and hay with blankets were placed outside, and to these 'beds' the less severely wounded were assigned. It was evident that the medical department of the army had failed absolutely to send hospital supplies, or by this time they would have been landed. As it was, the surgeons turned to the Red Cross ship 'State of Texas' for help, and the supplies originally intended for the starving Cubans were sent ashore for our wounded.

"Miss Barton had been urged and advised to wait until the army opened and made the way safe to land supplies for reconcentrados and refugees.

But she had foreseen the situation to a certain degree and followed the army as quickly as possible— to wait for the emergency, rather than have the emergency wait for her. The 'State of Texas' was here a week before the attack on Santiago.

"While surgeons and nurses were probing for bullets and dressing wounds, a force of men on the Red Cross ship worked half the night getting out cots and blankets, food and bandages, and at daylight next morning the supplies were landed, taking advantage of the smooth sea between four and nine o'clock, as later in the day the high surf makes it extremely difficult for landings. There were six tables in the operating-tent and eight surgeons. In twenty-four hours the surgeons had operated upon and dressed the wounds of 475 men. Four Red Cross sisters, trained nurses, assisted the surgeons. They were Sister Bettina, wife of Dr. Lesser, surgeon-in-chief of the Red Cross; Sister Minna, Sister Isabel, and Sister Blanche. Their knowledge of surgery, skill, and nerve were a revelation to the army surgeons. These young women, all under thirty, went from one operating-table to another, and, whatever was the nature of the wound or complication, proved equal to the emergency.

"In the Red Cross Hospital, across the way,

Sister Anna was in charge of the sick men, turned over to the Red Cross two days before, when army surgeons with troops were all ordered to the front. With 475 wounded men to feed there was not a camp-kettle to be found in which gruel could be prepared, coffee made or anything cooked, not a kettle of any sort to be furnished by the army. The whole camp outfit at Tampa in the way of cooking utensils must have been left behind.

"But there was an overruling Providence when the 'State of Texas' was loaded for Cuba. So far everything needed has been found in the hold of this old ship, which deserves to have and will have a credit page in the history of the war in Cuba. There were kettles, charcoal braziers, and cooking utensils carried over to the Red Cross Hospital. To prepare gruel, rice, coffee, and various other proper and palatable dishes for forty or fifty sick men by the slow process of a charcoal brazier, tea-kettle, and boiler is by no means easy cooking. But to prepare food for 475 wounded men, some of whom had had nothing to eat for twenty-four hours, cooking over a little charcoal pot is something that one must take a 'hand in' to fully appreciate.

"There was the feeling as if one were dazed and unnatural to hear American soldiers, men from comfortable homes, literally begging for ' just a spoonful of gruel.' The charcoal pot burned night and day, gallons of gruel were made and quantities of rice cooked until the greatest stress had passed. It was no time to stand on trained service, and everybody, man or woman, was ready to lend a hand.

" A striking feature of the first day's engagement was the number of men wounded in the head, arm, and upper part of the body. Some of these cases, the most serious, were taken into the Red Cross Hospital, where they received the most skilful and gentle nursing.

" Two days' steady strain began to show on the Sisters.

" The strain had been the greater because there were no facilities for anything like a regular meal short of the ship, reached by a long, hard tramp in the sand, then a row over the tossing waves. But nobody thought of meals. The one thing was to feed and nurse the 500 wounded and sick men. Human endurance, however, has its limit, and unless the Sisters could get a little rest they would give out. I went on duty for twenty-four hours, at night, with the assistance of one man, taking care of forty patients, fever, measles, and dysentery cases, and half a dozen badly wounded men.

Among the latter was Captain Mills, of the First Cavalry, and William Clark, a colored private in the Twenty-fifth Infantry, regulars. They were brought over from the hospital tents and placed on cots out on the little porch, where there was just room to pass between the cots.

"Their wounds were very similar—in the head —and of such a character as to require cool applications to the eyes constantly. Ice was scarce and worth its weight in gold, for the lives of these men as well as others depended chiefly on cool applications to the eyes, with as uniform temperature as possible. We had one small piece of ice, carefully wrapped in a blanket. There never was a small piece of ice that went so far. If I were to tell the truth about it nobody would believe me.

"Never in my whole life, I think, have I wished for anything so much as I wished for plenty of ice that night. It was applied by chipping in small bits, laid in thin, dry cotton cloth, folded over in just the right size and flat, to place across the eyes and forehead, enough of it to be cold, but not heavy, on the wounds.

"The ears of the sick are strangely acute. Whenever the sick men heard the sound of chipping ice they begged for ice-water; even the smallest bit of ice in a cup of water was begged with an eagerness that was pitiful. I felt conscience-smitten. But it was a question of saving the eyes of the wounded men, and there was no other way. To make the ice last till morning I stealthily chipped it off so the sick men would not hear the sound.

"At midnight a surgeon came over from his tent ward with a little piece of ice not larger than his hand. I do not know his name, but it does not matter, it is inscribed above. 'This is all we can spare,' he said. 'Take it. You must keep those wounds cool at all hazards. I have another case very like these—a man wounded in the head. I want to bring him over here, where he will be sure of exactly the same nursing. His life depends on the care he gets in the next twenty-four hours. Have you a vacant cot?'

"There was not a vacant cot, but we could make room for one on the porch if he could find the cot. He thought he could, and went back, taking the precious piece of ice that he really needed more than we did. In the course of a half hour the surgeon returned to say it was impossible to get a cot anywhere, and the wounded man must be left where he was in the tent, at least until morning.

"And so it went on through the long night— the patient suffering of the sick men, the heroism of the wounded, all fearing to give any trouble,

143

desiring not to do so, and grateful for the smallest attention.

"The courage that faces death on the battlefield or calmly awaits it in the hospital is not a courage of race or color. Two of the bravest men I ever saw were here, almost side by side on the little porch—Captain Mills and Private Clark— one white, the other black. They were wounded almost at the same time, and in the same way. The patient suffering and heroism of the black soldier was fully equal to that of the Anglo-Saxon. It was quite the same, the gentleness and appreciation. They were a study, these men so widely apart in life, but here strangely close and alike on the common ground of duty and sacrifice. They received precisely the same care; each fed like a child, for with their bandaged eyes they were as helpless as blind men. When the ice-pads were renewed on Captain Mills's eyes the same change was made on Private Clark's eyes. There was no difference in their beds or food. Neither uttered a word of complaint. The nearest to a regret expressed by Captain Mills was a heavy sigh, followed by the words: 'Oh, we were not ready. Our army was not prepared.'

"Of himself he talked cheerfully, strong, and hopeful. 'I think I shall go home with the sight of one eye,' he said. That was all.

"In the early part of the night he was restless, his brain was active, cool, and brave as he might be. The moonlight was very bright, a flood of silver, seen only in the tropics. Hoping to divert him I said: 'The moonlight is too bright, captain. I will put up a paper screen so you can get to sleep.'

"He realized at once the absurdity and the ludicrous side, and with an amused smile replied: 'But you know I can't see the moonlight.'

"I said it was time to get more ice for his head and half stumbled across the porch, blinded by tears. When told who his nearest neighbor was, Captain Mills expressed great sympathy for Private Clark and paid a high tribute to the bravery of the colored troops and their faithful performance of duty.

"Private Clark talked but little. He would lie apparently asleep until the pain in his head became unbearable. Then he would try to sit up, always careful to keep the ice-pad on his eyes over the bandage.

"'What can I do for you, Clark?' I would ask, anxious to relieve his pain.

"'Nothing, thank you,' he would answer. 'It's very nice and comfortable here. But it's only the misery in my head—the misery is awful.'

" Poor fellow! there was never a moan, merely a little sigh now and then, but always that wonderful patience that seemed to me not without a touch of divine philosophy, complete acceptance.

" I have mentioned these two men, not as exceptional in bravery, but to illustrate the rule of heroism, and because they were among the patients under my immediate care that night. It was a strange night picture—a picture that could never be dimmed by time but live through all the years of one's life.

" After midnight a restful atmosphere pervaded the hospital and the blessing of sleep fell upon the suffering men, one by one. In the little interval of repose I dropped into an old chair on the porch, looked away to the beautiful mountains sharply outlined in the moonlight, and the sea like waves of silver, the camp on the shore; near by thirty or forty horses standing motionless. Then the hospital tents, with now and then the flickering light of a candle; in the background the cliffs, with here and there a Spanish blockhouse. Over all the tragedy of life and death, the pain and sorrow, there was the stillness of a peaceful night—a stillness broken only by the sound of the surf brought back on the cool breeze, the cool, refreshing breeze, for which we all thanked God."

146

Later on, as will be remembered, Miss Jennings went North—a volunteer nurse on the transport Seneca. The brave men whose lives hung in the balance that night—with little hope that, if life were spared, they would ever see again—recovered, but each with the loss of an eye. After a long furlough Private Clark returned to his regiment. Captain Mills, now General Mills, is the Superintendent of the West Point Military Academy.

Three times in the first week I went over those terrible roads from the front to Siboney and return. Arriving at Siboney late one night, there was no way I could get on board the State of Texas and I was obliged to remain on shore. The Postmaster insisted that I occupy a room in the building used for a post-office. Such a courtesy could not be refused, and against all feeling of acquiescence, and with a dread as if there were something wrong about it, I allowed myself to be helped out of the wagon and entered the house. The Postmaster sat down and talked with me a little while. I thought he seemed ill. I had never met him before, but my heart went out in sympathy

147

for him. I feared I was taking his room, although
he did not admit it.

I was shown into a room where there was a cot,
a table, and a candle without a stick, burning upon
the table. The men went outside and laid down
upon the steps for the night. I laid down upon
the cot, but it was impossible for me to remain
there. Something constantly warned me to leave
it. I got up, went to the door, looked out upon
the night and darkness, and waited for the gray
of the morning. I went out and stood upon the
beach beside the sea and waited more and more,
until finally some of the men appeared, and I went
with them down to the water.

Six days later they told me that the rightful
occupant of the cot—the Postmaster, who had
seemed so ill—had died of a fever raging here that
they called "yellow fever." I had occupied his
cot. I wonder who it was that so continually
warned me that night to keep away from that room,
away from the cot, away from all connected with
it? "Yellow fever" was not then talked of. Did
some one tell me? I do not know—but something
told me.

The negotiations between General Shafter and the Spanish army at Santiago were going on. The flag of truce, that threatened every day to come down, still floated. The Spanish soldiers had been led by their officers to believe that every man who surrendered—and the people as well—would be butchered whenever the city should fall and the American troops should come in. But when General Shafter commenced to send back convoys of captured Spanish officers, their wounds dressed, and carefully placed on stretchers, borne under flags of truce to the Spanish lines at Santiago, and set down at the feet of General Toral, and when in astonishment that officer learned the object of the flag of truce and sent companies of his soldiers to form in line and present arms, while the cortege of wounded were borne through by American troops, a lesson was learned that went far toward the surrender of that city.

I happen to know that it was not without some very natural home criticism that General Shafter persisted in his course in the face of the time-honored custom of " hostages." One can readily understand that the voluntary giving up of

prisoners—officers at that—in view of an impend-
ing battle, might seem in the light of old-time
army usages a waste, to characterize it by no
harder term. It is possible that none of the officers
in that field had ever read the Articles of the Treaty
of Geneva, or fully recalled that the treaty had become a law, or that their commander was acting
in full accord with its wise and humane principles.

By this time the main talk of the camp was
" yellow fever." It was soon discovered by the
medical authorities that, from there having been
at first one case of fever, there were now one hundred and sixteen, and that a fever camp would
probably be made there, and the wounded gotten
away. It was advisable then that we return to our
ship and attempt, as far as possible, to hold that
free from contagion. I was earnestly solicited to
do this, in view of what was expected of our ship,
and of what was expected of us, that we not only
protect ourselves but our cargo and ship from all
contamination and even suspicion.

I faithfully promised to do so, and again called
for an army wagon, leaving all supplies that were
useful for the men in camp—sending to El Caney

what was most needed there—and taking only our personal effects, started for Siboney. In less than twenty minutes the rain was pouring on us and for two hours it fell as if from buckets. The water was from a foot and a half to two feet deep in the road as we passed along. At one time our wagon careened, the mules were held up, and we waited to see whether it should go over or could be brought out, the water a few inches only from the top of the lower side. It was scarcely possible for us to stir, hemmed in as we were, but the men from the other wagons sprang to our wheels, hanging in the air on the upper side, and we were simply saved by an inch.

But like other things, this cleared away. We came into Siboney about three o'clock, in a bright glare of sunshine, to find the town entirely burned —all buildings gone or smoking—and a " yellow fever " hospital established a mile and a half out from Siboney.

All effort was made to hold our ship free from suspicion. The process of reasoning leading to the conclusion that a solid cargo, packed in tight boxes in the hold of a ship, anchored at sea, could become infected in a day from the land or a passing individual, is indeed an intricate process. But we had some experience in this direction. Captain McCalla, in his repeated humane attempts to feed the refugees around Guantanamo, had called again for a hundred thousand rations, saying that if we could bring them to him soon he could get them to the starving people in the woods. We lost no time, but got the food out and started with it in the night. On reaching Guantanamo we were met some distance out, called to, and asked if any one on our ship had been on shore at Siboney within four days; if so, our supplies could not be received. We took them away, leaving the starving to perish.

The constantly recurring news of the surrender of Santiago was so well established that we drew anchor, came up to the flag-ship, and sent the following letter to Admiral Sampson:

" State of Texas,
" *July* 16, 1898.
" ADMIRAL SAMPSON, Commanding U. S. Fleet off Santiago, Flag-Ship New York.

"Admiral: It is not necessary for me to explain to you my errand, nor its necessity; both your good

152

head and heart divine it more clearly than any words of mine can represent.

"I send this to you by one of our men who can tell all you wish to know. Mr. John Elwell has resided and done mercantile and shipping business in Santiago for the last seven years; is favorably known to all its people; has in his possession the keys of the best warehouses and residences in the city, to which he is given welcome by the owners. He is the person appointed four months ago to help distribute this food, and did so with me until the blockade. There seems to be nothing in the way of getting our twelve hundred tons of food into a Santiago warehouse and giving it intelligently to the thousands who *need* and *own* it. I have twenty good helpers with me. The New York committee is urging the discharge of the State of Texas, which has been raised in price to four hundred dollars a day.

"If there is still more explanation needed, I pray you, Admiral, let me see you.

"Respectfuly and cordially,
"CLARA BARTON."

These were anxious days. While the world outside was making up war history, we thought of little beyond the terrible needs about us; if Santiago had any people left, they must be in sore distress; and El Caney, with its thirty thousand homeless, perishing sufferers, how could they be reached?

On that Sunday morning, never to be forgotten, the Spanish fleet came out of Santiago Harbor, to meet death and capture. That afternoon Lieutenant Capehart, of the flag-ship, came on board with the courteous reply of Admiral Sampson, that if we would come alongside the New York he would put a pilot on board. This was done, and we moved on through waters we had never traversed; past Morro Castle, long, low, silent, and grim; past the wrecks of the Spanish ships on the right; past the Merrimac in the channel. We began to realize that we were alone, of all the ships about the harbor there were none with us. The stillness of the Sabbath was over all. The gulls sailed and flapped and dipped about us. The lowering summer sun shot long golden rays athwart the green hills on either side and tinged the water calm and still. The silence grew oppressive as we glided along with scarce a ripple. We saw on the right as the only moving thing, a long, slim yacht dart out from among the bushes and steal its way up half-hidden in the shadows. Suddenly it was overtaken by either message or messenger, and like a collared hound glided back as if it had never been.

Leaning on the rail, half lost in reverie over the strange, quiet beauty of the scene, the thought suddenly burst upon me—are we really going into Santiago, and alone? Are we not to be run out, and wait aside, and salute with dipping colors, while the great battle-ships come up with music and banners and lead the way?

As far as the eye could reach no ship was in sight. Was this to remain so? Could it be possible that the commander who had captured a city declined to be the first to enter, that he would hold back his flag-ship and himself, and send forward and first a cargo of food on a plain ship, under direction of a woman? Did our commands, military or naval, hold men great enough of soul for such action? It must be true, for the spires of Santiago rise before us, and turning to the score of companions beside me I ask: " Is there any one here who will lead the Doxology?" In an instant the full rich voice of Enola Gardner rang out: " Praise God from whom all blessings flow." By that time the chorus was full, and the tears on many a face told more plainly than words how genuine was that praise, and when in response to a second suggestion " My Country 'Tis of Thee " swelled out on the evening air in the farewell rays of the setting sun, the State of Texas was nearing the dock, and quietly dropping her anchor she lay there through the silence of the night in un-disputed possession, facing a bare wind-swept wharf and the deserted city of Santiago.

Daybreak brought quiet to an end. The silence was no longer oppressive. A hundred and twenty stevedores lined up on the wharf for work and breakfast. The dock had tracks, and trucks run-ning to its open warehouses. Boxes, barrels, and bales, pitched out of that ship, thrown onto the trucks and wheeled away, told the story of better days to come. It was something to see the lank, brawny little army of stevedores take their first breakfast in line, alongside of the ship.

Later in the day the flag-ship brought Admiral Sampson and Admiral Schley, who spent several hours with us. They had every opportunity to see how our work was done, and if we were equal to unloading our ship. When they were about to leave Admiral Sampson was asked what orders or directions he had for us. He replied: " You need no directions from me, but if any one troubles you let me know."

The amiable pleasantries of these two gallant officers during that visit are a pleasure to recall. As I was, at an opportune moment, attempting to express my appreciation and thanks to Admiral Sampson for the courtesy of allowing us to precede him into Santiago, Admiral Schley, with that *naïveté* and apt turn of expression so characteristic of him, in a half undertone side-remark, cautioned me with " Don't give him too much credit, Miss Barton; he was not quite sure how clear the channel might be. Remember that was a trial trip."

How sadly the recollection of that pleasant, memorable day has since recurred to me; brave, gallant brothers in arms, and in heart; knowing only a soldier's duty; each holding his country's honor first, his own last; its glory his glory, and

157

for himself seeking nothing more. Ah, people, press, and politics! How deal ye with your servants?

A message was received from General Shafter, who telegraphed from his headquarters: " The death rate at El Caney is terrible; can you send food? " The answer was to send the thirty thousand refugees of El Caney at once back to Santiago; we were there and could feed them; that the State of Texas had still twelve hundred tons of supplies.

The thirty thousand inhabitants of Santiago had been driven to El Caney, a village designed for five hundred. In two days all were called back and fed, ten thousand the first day, twenty thousand the second. Then came our troops, and Santiago was lived and is remembered. Its hospitals, the ante-chamber to Montauk, are never to be forgotten.

A general committee was formed, the city districted into sections, with a commissioner for each district, selected by the people themselves living there. Every family or person residing within the city was supplied by the commissioner of that district, and all transient persons were fed at the kitchens, the food being provided by the Red Cross.

The discharge of the cargo of the State of Texas commenced at six o'clock Monday morning, July 18th. One hundred and twenty-five stevedores were employed and paid in food issued as rations. Four days later the discharge was completed.

Although the army had entered the city during the latter part of that time, there had been no confusion, no groups of disorderly persons seen, no hunger in the city more than in ordinary times. We had done all that could be done to advantage at that time in Santiago. The United States troops had mainly left. The Spanish soldiers were coming in to their waiting ships, bringing with them all the diseases that unprovided and uncleanly camps would be expected to hold in store. Five weeks before we had brought into Santiago all the cargo of the State of Texas excepting the hospital supplies, which had been used the month previous among our own troops at Siboney, General Shafter's front, and El Caney during the days of fighting.

These were the last days of General Shafter in Santiago, who was, as he had at all times been, the kind and courteous officer and gentleman. General Wood, who was made Governor of the Province of Santiago upon the day of surrender—alert, wise, and untiring, with an eye single to the good of all—toiled day and night.

The State of Texas steamed away to its northern home. Peace and plenty came. The reconcentrados we went in search of were never reached. To those who could not withstand, Heaven came. To those who could, *Cuba Libre.*

Later on, general efforts were made for the protection of the thousands of orphans over the island, in which efforts the Red Cross joined. But the people of Cuba solved the question themselves—by a general adoption in their own homes—and orphanages in Cuba became a thing of the past.

Thus our work on that distressful field closed, after nearly two years of such effort as one would never desire to repeat. The financial management of that field, so far as the Red Cross was concerned, was done under the attorneyship of the Central Cuban Relief Committee of New York, whose reports are models of accuracy and accountability, and to which any person desiring information may be referred.

Cuba was a hard field, full of heart-breaking memories. It gave the first opportunity to test the cooperation between the government and its supplemental handmaiden, the Red Cross. That these relations might not have been clearly understood at this initial date may well be appreciated, but that time and experience will remedy this may be confidently hoped.

Through all our discouragements the steady hand and calm approval of our great head of the army and navy was our solace and our strength. And when at length it was all over, his hand could trace for his message to his people the following testimonial, what need had one even to remember past discouragements, however great? It was as if the hand of the martyr had set its undying seal upon the brow of the American Red Cross. What greater justification could it have? What greater riches could it crave?

"In this connection it is a pleasure for

161

me to mention in terms of cordial appreciation the timely and useful work of the American Red Cross, both in relief measures preparatory to the campaigns, in sanitary assistance at several of the camps of assemblage, and, later, under the able and experienced leadership of the president of the society, Miss Clara Barton, on the fields of battle and in the hospitals at the front in Cuba. Working in conjunction with the governmental authorities and under their sanction and approval, and with the enthusiastic cooperation of many patriotic women and societies in the various States, the Red Cross has fully maintained its already high reputation for intense earnestness and ability to exercise the noble purposes of its international organization, thus justifying the confidence and support which it has received at the hands of the American people. To the members and officers and all who aided them in their philanthropic work, the sincere and lasting gratitude of the soldiers and the public is due and freely accorded.

"In tracing these events we are constantly reminded of our obligations to the Divine Master for His watchful care over us, and His safe guidance, for which the nation makes reverent acknowledgment and offers humble prayers for the continuance of His favors."—FROM PRESIDENT McKINLEY'S MESSAGE TO CONGRESS, DECEMBER 6, 1898.

IX

THIS time there was no murmur in the air, no warning of approaching danger. Even the watchful press, that knows so much before it ever happens, slumbered quiet and deep, till the hissing wires shrieked the terrifying word—Galveston.

Then we learned that, as at Port Royal, the sea had overleaped its bounds and its victims by thousands were in its grasp.

In all the land no one slept then. To us it was the clang of the fire-bell, and the drop of the harness. The Red Cross clans commenced to gather.

In two days a little coterie of near a dozen left Washington under escort of the competent agency of the New York World, which had on the first day telegraphed that it would open a subscription for the relief of Galveston, and would be glad to send all supplies and money received to the Red Cross,

164

if its president, Miss Clara Barton, would go and distribute it. It was the acceptance of this generous offer that had brought to the station in Washington the escort; and a palace-car, provided with all comforts for the journey to Galveston, was under the management of the World's efficient correspondent and agent, Robert Adamson.

The direfulness of the news gathered as we proceeded on our journey, and delays were gotten over as quickly as possible. A detention of several hours in New Orleans gave opportunity for consultation with the officers of the Red Cross Society of that city, which had held its loyal ranks unbroken since 1882, and became a tower of strength in this relief. A day of waiting in Houston for a passage over the Gulf gave us a glimpse of what the encroachment had been on the mainland. We found the passage across to Galveston difficult, and with one night of waiting by the shore in almost open cars, at Texas City, we at length arrived in Galveston on the morning of the 15th of September.

Here again no description could adequately serve its purpose. The sea, with fury spent, had sullenly retired. The strongest buildings, half

standing, roofless and tottering, told what once
had been the make-up of a thriving city. But that
cordon of wreckage skirting the shore for miles it
seemed, often twenty feet in height, and against
which the high tide still lapped and rolled! What
did it tell? The tale is all too dreadful to recall—
the funeral pyre of at least five thousand human
beings. The uncoffined dead of the fifth part of a
city lay there. The lifeless bodies festering in the
glaring heat of a September sun told only too
fatally what that meant to that portion of the
city left alive. The streets were well-nigh im-
passable, the animals largely drowned, the working force of men diminished, dazed, and homeless.
The men who had been the fathers of the city, its
business and its wealth, looked on aghast at their
overwhelmed possessions, ruined homes, and, worse
than all, mourned their own dead.

Yet these men, to the number of thirty or
more, had, as one may say, pulled themselves together, and were even at that early date a relief
committee, holding their meetings at the wrecked
and half-ruined hotel, almost the only public house
left standing. To this hotel we also went and re-

ported to the committee. To say that we were kindly and gratefully received by them says nothing that would satisfy either ourselves or them.

The conditions were so new to them that it was a relief to meet persons who had seen such things before. We were asked not only to act with them, but to assume charge of the administration of relief. This, of course, we would not do, but that we would meet with, counsel, and aid them in every way in our power, is needless to affirm. That we did do this, through every day of our stay of three months, not only our own conviction, but the unasked and unexpected testimony of both Galveston and the Legislature of the State of Texas, go to assure.

On the third day after our arrival we were joined by Mr. Stephen E. Barton, President of the former Central Cuban Relief Committee, and Mr. Fred L. Ward, its competent secretary, who became our secretary from the time of his arrival until the close of the field, continuing until after our return to headquarters and settling the last account. Not only the thanks of the Red Cross are due for his faithful, painstaking work, but his

name is still a household word through the score
of counties skirting the shore on the mainland of
Texas.

It may be interesting to readers to know what is
done first, or just how a relief party commence
under circumstances like that. A few words will
give an outline. First the ground must be overlooked and conditions learned. This is not easy
when it is remembered that broken houses, cars,
wagons, church steeples, and grand pianos were
liable to be encountered in the middle of the leading
streets, themselves buried three feet in the coarse
black sand, brought in by the great tidal wave.

Nevertheless, a building must be found in which
to store and distribute the supplies that would immediately come. How needful these supplies would
be can be inferred when it is recalled that scores of
persons came alive out of that wreck, with simply
the band of a shirt or a night-dress held by its
button about the neck as the only reminder that
ever a cover of clothing had been theirs.

A little meeting of my assistants early held assigned each to his duty and his place. A warehouse, fortunately still intact, was generously sup-

plied by Mr. John Sealy. Major James A. McDowell, with the experience of this branch of Red Cross work from Johnstown down, and the record of twenty-six battles in the old civil war, was placed in charge. Here is one of the scenes given by a casual eye-witness:

A poor feeble-looking man, with scant clothing, enters the warehouse and waits. "Hello there," calls the observant major—with his Grand Army button—overhauling clothes for the visitor. "But, major, I was a Confederate soldier." "Lord bless your poor suffering soul, what difference does that make? Here, this will suit you."

It was thought advisable by some of the party to establish an orphanage, which was done and carried through, regardless of the common-sense idea that few children would survive, when the parents were drowned. And so it proved, although the work was faithfully administered.

Homes must be made, lumber obtained, and houses built. The Red Cross sent out the appeal for lumber and aided in the work of shelter.

Mrs. Fannie B. Ward was placed in charge of a special clothing department. Need I remind thoughtful readers that in a disaster like that, where people of affluence, culture, and position are in a night bereft of all, one of the cruelest features might be to go to the open boxes of a relief station for clothing, such as never before worn, and could not be asked for through the choking tears. In all humanity these cases must be properly, respectfully, and discreetly met, as one lady could meet another in distress.

No more vivid picture of the conditions by which we were surrounded can be imagined than the following extract from Mrs. Ward's report:

"Just seven days after the storm we found ourselves stranded at Texas City, on the mainland opposite Galveston Island, waiting for transportation across the six-mile stretch of water. Bridges had been swept away, and new sand-bars thrown up in the bay; floating roofs and timbers impeded navigation, and the only method of communication between the mainland and Galveston was one poor little ferry-boat, which had to feel her now dangerous way very cautiously, by daylight only. She had also to carry nearly a quarter of her capacity in soldiers to prevent her being swamped by waiting crowds of people, frantic to learn the fate of their friends on the island. Each trip to the mainland, the boat came filled with refugees from the city of doom—the sick, the maimed, the sorrowing —many with fearful bodily injuries inflicted by the storm, and others with deeper wounds of grief; —mothers whose babies had been torn from their arms, children whose parents were missing, fathers whose entire families were lost—a dazed and tearless throng, such as Danté might have met in his passage through Inferno. These were dumped by thousands on the sandy beach at Texas City, and then conveyed by rail to Houston, to be cared for by the good people of that city, who, notwithstanding their own grievous losses, were doing noble work for their stricken neighbors.

"Of Texas City—a flourishing town of four or five thousand houses—nothing remained but heaps of bricks and splintered wood, sodden bales of cotton and bits of household furniture, scattered over the plain; not a standing habitation within miles, nor any shelter for the crowds above-mentioned, except two or three hospital-tents, hastily set up for the sick and wounded, but inadequate for their

171

accommodation. What was our dismay when told
that here we must remain at least twenty-four
hours, for the return of the boat! However, we
were better off, even physically, than most of the
waiting crowd, though weariness of the flesh
amounted to actual suffering, after more than fifty
hours' travel. As a special courtesy to Miss Barton, the railway company left a car to shelter her
during the night. Luxurious Pullmans did not
abound at Texas City, and this was the shabbiest
of day-coaches, equipped with few 'modern conveniences.' But this was no time to think of personal comfort, on the threshold of so much misery;
and who could murmur when the head of our little
company set such an heroic example of patience.
I have seen her in many trying situations, that
threatened the fortitude and endurance of the
strongest—and have yet to hear the first word of
complaint from her lips. She smilingly 'bunked'
upon two seats laid together—compared to which,
for softness, the *penitente's* slab of stone would be
as 'downy beds of ease'—and encouraged her
companions to do the same. Hunger and thirst
would also have been our portion, had it not been

for a Salvation Army Corps encamped in the vicinity, and the Relief Train of the Philadelphia North American, stranded like ourselves. Thanks to those good Samaritans, we dined and breakfasted on tinned beef, bread and coffee; and what more could good soldiers require?

" That night in Texas City will be long remembered. Sleep was out of the question—stretched on those cross-bars, like St. Lawrence on his gridiron. Soldiers patrolled the beach, not only to prevent a stampede of the boat, but to protect both the quick and the dead from fiends in human guise, who prowled the devastated region, committing atrocities too horrible to name. All night the steady tramp, tramp, of the guard sounded beneath the car-windows, while at either door stood two sentinels, muskets on shoulders. Skies of inky blackness, studded with stars of extraordinary brilliancy, seemed to bend much nearer the earth than at the North; and the Great Dipper hung low on the horizon—for only just across the Gulf it disappears to give place to the Southern Cross. Myriads of big, bright fire-flies, resembling balls of flame, flitted restlessly over the plain, like the

173

disembodied souls whose homes were here one short
week before, searching for their scattered treasures.
Over on Galveston Island, a long line of flame,
mounting to the heavens, marked the burning of
ruined homes and corpses; while other fires, in all
directions on the mainland, told of similar ghastly
cremations. At one time I counted twenty-three
of these fires, not including those on the island.
Early in the morning a strange odor drew attention
to a fresh funeral-pyre, only a few rods away,
around the horse-shoe curve of the shore. We
were told that thirty bodies, found since daybreak
in the immediate vicinity, were being consumed in
it. That peculiar smell of burning flesh, so sick-
ening at first, became horribly familiar within the
next two months, when we lived in it and breathed
it, day after day.

" We found the situation in Galveston infinitely
worse than had been described. The most sensa-
sational accounts of the yellowest journals fell far
short of the truth—simply because its full horror
was beyond the power of words to portray. Figures and statistics can give little idea of the results
of such an appalling calamity; and to this day,

people at a distance have no realization of the unutterable woe which our Red Cross band of less than a dozen, strove to alleviate. We arrived on the eighth day after the tragedy, in which upward of ten thousand lives went suddenly out in storm and darkness; and the survivors were just beginning to realize the extent of their losses.

" At first they seemed stunned to partial insensibility by the very magnitude of their grief—as a man who has been mangled almost unto death in a railroad disaster is said to be oblivious to pain. Dead citizens lay by thousands amid the wreck of their homes, and raving maniacs searched the *débris* for their loved ones, with the organized gangs of workers. Corpses, dumped by barge-loads into the Gulf, came floating back to menace the living; and the nights were lurid with incinerations of putrefying bodies, piled like cord-wood, black and white together, irrespective of age, sex, or previous condition. At least four thousand dwellings had been swept away, with all their contents, and fully half of the population of the city was without shelter, food, clothes, or any of the necessaries of life. Of these, some were living in tents; others crowded in

175

with friends hardly less unfortunate; many half-crazed, wandering aimlessly about the streets, and the story of their sufferings, mental and physical, is past the telling. Every house that remained was a house of mourning. Of many families every member had been swept away. Even sadder were the numerous cases where one or two were left out of recently happy households; and saddest of all was the heart-breaking suspense of those whose friends were numbered among the 'missing.'

"We find it hard enough to lay away our dead in consecrated ground, with all the care and tenderness that love can suggest, where we may water the sacred spot with our tears and place upon it the flowers they loved in life; but never to know whether their poor bodies were swallowed by the merciless Gulf, or fed to the fishes with those grewsome barge-loads, or left above ground to become an abomination in the nostrils of the living, or burned in indiscriminate heaps with horses and dogs and the mingled ashes scattered to the winds—must indeed have been well-nigh unbearable. No wonder there were lunatics in Galveston, and unnumbered cases of nervous prostration.

176

" After weeks had passed and two thousand men, aided by several hundred teams, had partially reduced the mountain of wreckage, cremation fires yet burned continuously—fed not only by human bodies, but by thousands of carcasses of domestic animals. By that time, in the hot, moist atmosphere of the latitude, decomposition had so far advanced that the corpses—which at first were decently carried in carts or on stretchers, then shoveled upon boards or blankets—had finally to be scooped up with pitchforks, in the hands of negroes, kept at their awful task by the soldiers' bayonets. And still the ' finds ' continued, at the average rate of seventy a day. The once beautiful driving beach was strewn with mounds and trenches, holding unrecognized and uncoffined victims of the flood; and between this improvised cemetery and a ridge of *débris*, three miles long and in places higher than the houses had been, a line of cremation fires poisoned the air.

" I think it was during our sixth week in Galveston, when, happening to pass one of these primitive crematories, I stopped to interview the man in charge. Boards, water-soaked mattresses,

177

rags of blankets and curtains, part of a piano, baby-carriages, and the framework of sewing-machines, piled on top, gave it the appearance of a festive bonfire, and only the familiar odor betrayed its purpose.

" 'Have you burned any bodies here?' I inquired. The custodian regarded me with a stare that plainly said, 'Do you think I am doing this for amusement?' and shifted his quid from cheek to cheek before replying.

" 'Ma'am,' said he, 'this 'ere fire's been goin' on more'n a month. To my knowledge, upwards of sixty bodies have been burned in it—to say nothin' of dogs, cats, hens, and three cows.'

" 'What is in there now?' I asked.

" 'Wa'al,' said he meditatively, 'it takes a corpse several days to burn all up. I reckon thar's a couple of dozen of 'em—jest bones, you know—down near the bottom. Yesterday we put seven on top of this 'ere pile, and by now they are only what you might call baked. To-day we have been working over there (pointing to other fires a quarter of a mile distant), where we found a lot of 'em, 'leven under one house. We have put only two in

178

here to-day. Found 'em just now, right in that
puddle.'

" ' Could you tell me who they are? ' I asked.

" 'Lord! No,' was the answer. ' We don't look
at 'em any more'n we have to, else we'd been dead
ourselves before to-day. One of these was a colored man. They are all pretty black, now; but
you can tell 'em by the kinky hair. He had nothin'
but an undershirt and one shoe. The other was a
woman; young, I reckon. 'Tenny rate she was tall
and slim and had lots of long brown hair. She
wore a blue silk skirt and there was a rope tied
around her waist, as if somebody had tried to save
her.'

" Taking a long pole he prodded an air-hole
near the center of the smoldering heap, from which
now issued a frightful smell, that caused a hasty
retreat to the windward side. The withdrawal of
the pole was followed by a shower of charred bits
of bone and singed hair. I picked up a curling,
yellow lock and wondered, with tears, what mother's
hand had lately caressed it.

" ' That's nothin',' remarked the fireman. ' The
other day we found part of a brass chandelier, and

179

wound all around it was a perfect mop of long, silky hair—with a piece of skin, big as your two hands, at the end of it. Some woman got tangled up that way in the flood and jest na'cherly scalped.'

" I mention these incidents merely to show some of the conditions that had to be met. The most we could do for the grief-stricken survivors was to mitigate in some degree their bodily distress. The world knows how generously the whole country responded to the call—how contributions came pouring in by trainloads and shiploads, consigned to the Red Cross. To distribute all this bounty judiciously was a herculean task—and our working force was very small. The ladies and gentlemen of Galveston who had suffered less than their neighbors, formed themselves into committees, which opened relief stations in the several wards; and through these channels the bulk of supplies was issued. If mistakes were made, it was not from lack of faithful endeavor on the part of the distributers; and let us hope that the errors, if any, were all on the side of too liberal giving.

" Merely to sort over one carload of garments, so

as to make them immediately available—to put the infants' clothes in one department, the shoes in another, grown-up dresses in another, coats and trousers in another, underwear in another—was a work of time and strength; as the writer, who for a while was 'Mistress of the Robes,' can testify. From 7 A. M. till dark we toiled; and when at last we dragged ourselves back to the hotel, too wearied for anything but bed, 'tired Nature's sweet restorer' was hard to woo, because of aching feet and swollen muscles. But the experience was well worth it! Besides the joy of administering to the suffering, what we learned of human nature (mostly good, I am glad to say) would fill volumes. To be sure, there were shadows, as well as lights, in the picture. Greed and hypocrisy, jealousy, malice, and the reverse of Christian charity, came sometimes unpleasantly to the fore, to be offset by the magnificent generosity of the American nation, and the knowledge that in most quarters our efforts were appreciated. Most of us were unused to manual labor, and all had left comfortable homes— some at considerable financial sacrifice of well-salaried positions, not for earthly gain or self-aggrandizement, but from pure love of the splendid cause of the Cross of Geneva.

"In that Rag Fair department of old clothes, the ludicrous and pathetic called for an equal blending of smiles and tears. It seemed as if every household, from Maine to California, from the St. Lawrence to the Rio Grande, had rummaged its attics for the flood sufferers. Merchants delivered themselves of years' accumulations of shop-worn goods—streaked, faded, of fashions long gone by —but a great deal better than nothing for the destitute. There were at least a million shirt-waists, all thin and summery, though cold winter was at hand, when frequent 'northers' chill the very marrow in one's bones, and ice and snow are not unknown on Galveston Island. There was an-other million of 'Mother Hubbard' wrappers, all of the sleaziest print and scrimpest pattern, with inch-wide hems at bottom and no fastening to speak of—wrappers enough to disfigure every female in Southern Texas. Fancy a whole city full of women masquerading in those shapeless garments—the poorest of their class; and then remember that, a few years ago, the great and glorious State of

Pennsylvania found it necessary to pass a law—presumably for the peace of mind of her male citizens—forbidding the wearing of 'Mother Hubbards' in the street!

"One day there came to our warehouse a large case of beautiful, buttoned shoes, of the kind called 'Sorosis.' 'What a bonanza!' we thought, when that box was opened—and through our minds went trooping a procession of the shoeless feet we had longed to comfort. But behold! every blessed shoe of the one hundred and forty-four was for the left foot!

"There was an enormous box from a city laundry, containing the unclaimed 'washings' of many years—hundreds of waiters' aprons and cooks' caps, worn hotel towels and napkins, ragged shirts and collars—not a thing worth the lumber in the box, except as old linen for the hospitals. There was a great deal of bedraggled finery, than which nothing could have been less appropriate, when nine out of every ten women who applied for clothes, wanted plain black in which to mourn for their dead. And the hats and bonnets were of every shape and style within the memory of man! They were mostly so crushed in careless packing that to have worshiped them would have been no sin, according to Scripture, as they were no longer in the 'likeness of anything in the heavens above, or the earth beneath, or the waters under the earth.' There were workmen's blouses and overalls, evidently shed in haste, under a sudden impulse of generosity—plastered with grease, paint, and mortar, and odoriferous of that by which honest bread is said to be earned.

" Occasionally a box or barrel was found to contain garments disgracefully dirty and ragged, or dropping in pieces from the ravages of moths. Possibly the sending of such worthless trash produced in the hearts of the donors that comfortable feeling of lending to the Lord—but it was no use at our end of the line. What to do with it was a problem. The lowest plantation darky would regard the gift as an insult, and to burn even the filthiest rags would give rise to stories of wanton waste. So we hit upon an expedient which had been successfully employed in other fields—that of putting worthless articles in nice, clean barrels, rolling them out on the doorstep, and forgetting to bring them in at night; and every morning the barrels were found empty.

"In striking contrast to these few 'shadows' were such gifts as that of the New England girl, who sent a large, carefully packed satchel, accompanied by a letter, explaining that she was seventeen years of age, and had taken from her own wardrobe an outfit, intended for a flood-sufferer of about her own age, whom the clothes would fit. The satchel contained three good suits complete, from hat to hose—all that a girl would need—even veil, handkerchiefs and fan; and it is needless to add that they soon found their way to a most grateful young 'sufferer.' Here a poor widow divided her well-worn 'mourning' with some stranger sister-in-grief; there the bereaved mother brought out the treasured garments her little one had worn, for some happier mother who had lost only earthly possessions.

"Letters by hundreds were found in the packages, pertinent and impertinent, but all demanding answers. They were stuffed into old shoes and the linings of hats, cracked tea-pots and boxes of soap, combs and matches. Every small boys'

18　　　185

knickerbockers contained a note—generally of original spelling and laboriously written in large capi-
tals, from ' Tommy ' or ' Johnnie ' or ' Charley,'
asking a reply, telling all about the storm, from
the boy who should receive the gift. Sentimental
epistles from ladies were hidden in the pockets of
coats and trousers, inviting correspondence with
the future wearers; and billet-doux from disconsolate widowers, presumably beginning to ' take
notice,' were pinned to the raiment of deceased
wives. Such manifold phases have our poor human
nature! Happily there was another and far more
numerous class of letters, from charitable men and
women, offering to adopt children, or to assist in
any way in their power; from Sunday-school
classes and sewing societies and day-schools, enclosing small sums of money, or telling of gifts to
come. There was even a letter from an almshouse,
enclosing a check for eighty dollars, raised by
thirty aged pensioners, who gave up their only
luxuries—coffee, sugar, and tobacco—to swell the
fund for Galveston's relief. Another came from
the poor, forgotten negroes of the Carolina sea
islands, to whose assistance the Red Cross went,

after their disastrous floods a few years ago. Impelled by gratitude for the benefits then received, those simple-minded people contributed a surprising amount, considering their poverty. Truly, in heaven's reckoning those unselfish ' mites ' of the poor and lowly will count for as much as the millions given by the great cities.

" Notwithstanding the vast amount of old clothes that came to us, we were always particularly short of the most important articles of an outfit, such as underwear, respectable skirts and dresses, and shoes—except of extraordinary sizes, sent because unsalable. It frequently happened that, for days together, there was hardly a thing in stock fit for people of the better class. It must be remembered that we were not supplying tramps and beggars, nor the ordinary applicants for charity, but ladies and gentlemen, accustomed to the luxuries of life, whose possessions had been suddenly swept away. How could we offer those dreadful wrappers, or bedraggled finery, or soiled and ragged garments which our servants would despise, to ladies of taste, culture, and refinement, whom we had come to assist in their misfortune, not to insult? Therefore, in many cases, the only decent thing to do was to go out and buy what was needed, with some of those blessed contributions which bore the message, 'to be used at your own discretion.' That was Christian charity, pure and simple, in its most practical form. For example: A widow, of highest social standing and former wealth, lived with her three daughters in one of those ill-fated cottages near the beach, which was swept away with all its contents. Thus the four helpless women were left entirely destitute, even the clothes on their backs borrowed from neighbors a little less unfortunate. Friends in a Northern city wrote, offering them a home. Transportation could be easily provided, but the four must be fittted out for the journey. We searched the Rag Fair over, but found few suitable articles. Perhaps something better might come in by and by, next week, some other time; but for every hoped-for article were a hundred waiting applicants—and meanwhile those ladies must be supported until sent to their friends. To say nothing of their own feelings, and ours, we could not disgrace the Red Cross by sending that stately gray-haired mother and the three delicate young ladies out into the world equipped by our alleged bounty in scanty calico 'Mother Hubbards,' men's cow-hide brogans, and scare-crow headgear. So we picked out what would answer—here and there a garment which might be altered, the only pair of shoes in the place that came near to fitting one of the ladies, a bolt of unbleached muslin which they, themselves, could fashion into underclothes, and four disreputable old hats. The latter we gave to a local milliner to remodel and trim, simply but respectably. Then we went to the store and purchased shoes and other necessary articles, including enough inexpensive but serviceable cloth for four gowns and jackets, and employed a woman to make them.

"This was not extravagance, but good use of the money, all around:—for the poor little milliner whose shop had been destroyed and business ruined, whose children were then eating the bread of charity; and for the customless dressmaker, who was also a grievous sufferer by the flood, with younger sisters to support. We gave her the first work she had had for weeks, and her gratitude was good to see.

189

" As for merchants, who were all on the verge of failure, but making heroic efforts to keep afloat —Heaven knows we did them injury enough every day of our stay in Galveston, to be thankful for the privilege of occasionally becoming their patrons. Not only had they suffered immense losses by the storm, their stocks being practically ruined and customers gone—but who would buy, so long as the Red Cross had food and clothes to give away, without money and without price? Though ours is a noble and necessary work, it is never to the advantage of the local merchants, as a little reflection will show.

" Another case was that of a young woman, who, with an aged relative, was keeping a hotel in a near-by village, when the floods lifted their house from its foundations and ruined everything in it. Its four walls stood, however, and furnished shelter for all the houseless neighbors, who flocked in, naked and hungry, and with whom the generous girl divided her last garment and bit of food. Death also entered the family, twice within a few weeks—the last time leaving a sister's four half-grown children for this young woman to maintain.

190

Take them she must, because they had nowhere else to go. Finding her in terrible straits, without even clothes to wear to her sister's funeral, were we not justified in buying the heroic young woman a decent suit of black, besides sending her a box of food supplies? Why were we there, if not to exercise judgment in the matter of relief? If merely to distribute second-hand articles, without discrimination, we might have saved ourselves much peril and hardship by remaining at home, and sending the boxes down to take care of themselves.

"None of us will ever forget the grandniece of an ex-President of the United States—a handsome and imposing woman of middle age, traveled, educated, and evidently accustomed to the best society. She called one day at headquarters, and although she did not ask for aid, the truth came out in a heart-to-heart talk with Miss Barton that she had lost all in the storm and had not where to lay her head, nor food for the morrow; even the clothes she wore were not her own. Nobody living could put this lady on the pauper list, and none with a spark of human feeling could wish to wound her pride. Our honored President, who reads hearts as others do open books, clasped this unfortunate sister's hand—and left in it a bank-note—I do not know of what denomination, but let us hope it was not a small one. The look of surprise and gratitude that flashed over that woman's face was worth going far to see, as, speechless with emotion, the tears streaming down her cheeks, she turned away.

"One might go on multiplying incidents by the hour, did time permit. There were teachers to be fitted out with suitable clothes before the opening of the schools; boys and girls needing school-books and shoes, caps, and jackets; new-born babes to be provided, whose wardrobes, prepared in advance, had been swept away; mothers of families, destitute of the commonest conveniences of life, to whom the gift of a pan or kettle was a godsend; aged people, whose declining years must be comforted; invalids to be cheered with little luxuries. My greatest regret is that we had not hundreds of dollars to use for every one that was expended in these directions."

My stenographer, Miss Agnes Coombs, found her post by me, and sixty to eighty letters a day,

taken from dictation, made up the clerical round
of the office of the president. This duty fell in between attending the daily meetings of the relief
committee and receiving constant calls both in and
out of the city.

Our men made up their living-room at the warehouse. The few women remained at the hotel, the
only suitable place in the town.

Later on arrived a shipload of supplies from
the business people of New York, which were stored
with the Galveston committee, and we were asked
to aid in the distribution of these supplies, and to
a certain extent we did, but succeeded in organiz-
ing a committee of citizens, ladies and gentlemen,
to carry out and complete this distribution.

From lack of knowledge of the real conditions
of the disaster and its geographical extent, this
munificent donation had been assigned to the " Relief of Galveston," and thus, technically, Galveston
had no authority to administer a pound or a dollar
to any communities or persons outside of the pre-
cincts of the city proper. This left at least twenty
counties on the mainland on the other side of the
Gulf, some of which were as badly wrecked and

ruined as Galveston itself, without a possibility of the slightest benefit from this great, generous gift.

Seeing this pitiful and innocently unjust condition of affairs, the result of ignorance of relief work, undertaken with much zeal but scant knowledge and no experience, we sought a way to atone for the mistake, so far as we might be able.

Immediately closing our relief rooms in Galveston I had all Red Cross supplies shipped to Houston, and relief for the mainland opened there. These were farming districts, and I directed intelligent inquiry to be made as to what was most needed by the devastated farm lands and their owners. All was swept away—sometimes as far as forty miles back into the level country; often the soil itself was washed away, the home and all smaller animals destroyed, and no feed for the larger ones to subsist on. The poor farmers walked their desolated fields and wrung their hands.

It proved that this was the strawberry section of Southern Texas, and these were the strawberry growers that supplied the early berries to our Northern market. For miles not a plant was left

194

and no means to replant. This was reported to me on the first day's investigation, and also that if plants could be obtained and set within two weeks a half crop could be grown this year and the industry restored. That seemed a better occupation for these poor fellows than walking the ground and wringing their hands. The messenger was sent back at daybreak to ascertain how many plants would be needed to replant these lands, where they were accustomed to procure them, and what varieties were best adapted to their use.

That night brought again the messenger to say that a million and a half of plants would reset the lands and that their supply came from the nurseries in North Carolina, Illinois, Arkansas, and Louisiana. Directions were sent back to Mr. Ward to order the plants to be there in two weeks. This was done. Only thirty-eight thousand plants were injured in transit, and those were generously resupplied by the shippers. Within the two weeks this million and a half of strawberry plants were set. It was estimated that fully a third of a crop was realized that year, and it is safe to predict that one-half the readers of this little sketch will

195

partake of the fruits of these Red Cross relief strawberry fields this very springtime.

Other needs to a large amount were supplied by Mr. Ward, and we left no idle, wringing hands on the mainlands of Texas.

I had never left Galveston. Some other thoughtful reader may pitifully ask, what became of these miles of wreckage and the dead on the Galveston seashore?

At this distant day it may be safe to tell. I recall that at the time much criticism was indulged in.

All were burned.

The heat grew greater and the stench stronger every day. They tried to remove the *débris* and get the bodies out for burial. No human being could work in that putrefying mass. Previously had come the glorious thought of getting them into boats and shipping them a mile out to sea. With hopeful hearts this experiment was tried for one day. Alas! the night tide brought them all back to shore. The elements of earth and water had refused—what remained but fire? Openings in the long continuous lines were cut

196

through at given spaces, the fire engines set to play on the open, and the torch applied to the end of sections; thus a general conflagration of the city was prevented, and from day to day the pile diminished.

The stench of burning flesh permeated every foot of the city. Who could long withstand this? Before the end of three months there was scarcely a well person in Galveston. My helpers grew pale and ill, and even I, who have resisted the effect of so many climates, needed the help of a steadying hand as I walked to the waiting Pullman on the track, courteously tendered free of charge to take us away.

This is a tedious story; but if gone through, one has a little insight into the labor of a Red Cross field of relief. There are twenty in my recollection, and this was by no means the hardest or the most useful. They have been lived, but never told.

I beg my readers to bear in mind that this is not romance that I am writing, where I can place my characters in the best light and shape results at will, but history, with my personages still alive, ready to attest the reality of this statement. That

grand committee of Galveston relief—than whom
no nobler body of men I have ever met—are, I
hope, all yet alive to testify to the conditions and
statements made.

I have dedicated this little volume to the people
with whom, and for whom, have gone the willing
labors of twenty-five years—initial labors, untried
methods, and object lessons. Well or ill, they
have carried with them the best intentions and the
best judgment given for the purpose. Whatever
may betide or the future have in store for the little
work so simply commenced, so humbly carried on,
merely a helper with no thought of leadership, it
bears along with it the memories of pain assuaged,
hope revived, endeavor strengthened, and lives
saved.

To the noble sympathies of generous hearts these
results are due, and yet it is not in its past that
the glories or the benefits of the Red Cross lie, but
in the possibilities it has created for the future; in
the lessons it has taught; in the avenues to humane
effort it has opened, and in the union of beneficent
action between people and Government, when once
comprehended and effected, that shall constitute a

bulwark against the mighty woes sure to come sooner or later to all peoples and all nations.

To you—the people of America—this sacred trust is committed, in your hands the charge is laid. To none will your help ever be so precious as it has been to me, for in its proud growth and strength none will ever so need you.

Printed in the United States
137746LV00004B/10/A

9 780548 312834